Beating the
Dementia
Monster

Out of all the things I've lost, I miss my mind the most.

—Mark Twain

Beating the Dementia Monster

How I stopped the advance of cognitive impairment from Alzheimer's disease

David H. Brown

Beating the Dementia Monster: How I stopped the advance of cognitive impairment from Alzheimer's disease

ISBN 978-1981347117

Printed in USA

Dedication

This book is dedicated to the men and women of the Alzheimer's community—the researchers, the doctors and other health care workers, the caregivers, and the sufferers. Let us hope for a major breakthrough to bring an end to this terrible disease.

Table of Contents

Acknowledgements

In undertaking the project of writing this book, I needed to contend with the fact that I would discuss complex matters about which I was not an expert. Therefore, I relied heavily on several people who reviewed the manuscript and made important suggestions and corrections. All of them were greatly encouraging to me.

My first version needed a lot of work. The presentation was confused and very badly organized. I am deeply in debt to my wife Amy, my sister-in-law Carrie, and our friend Dr. Tae-Im Moon who reviewed it and made important suggestions. Oddly, working independently, they all came up with pretty much the same recommendations. (Or maybe that wasn't so odd.)

I appreciate the hard work and the patience of my son Aaron, the first sign of my strength, who performed the copy editing of the manuscript. He knows more than I do about where to put all of those commas, and I'm a slow learner.

I am indebted to my care team at Harborview Medical Center in Seattle. Aside from providing excellent medical care, they gave me many of the insights that I share in this book.

I am indebted to Dr. Vaishali Phatak who was my neuropsychologist at Harborview and is now at the University of Nebraska School of Medicine. Her review and comment on the manuscript were very helpful. (I also appreciate her kind words about my photography.)

I am indebted to Dr. Stuart Freeman who reviewed a late version of the manuscript and provided very helpful comments.

I appreciate the willingness of Dr. Moon to write the foreword.

My sister Renate provided wise counsel during the difficult but vitally important process of developing the cover design.

Jessica Ni, Kay Kaffer, and Shannon Douglas were instrumental in developing the final concept for the cover design.

Lastly, I am eternally grateful to the many family and friends who have been in prayer for me from the beginning of my adventure. Surely their prayers have been heard.

Foreword

In 2015, Dave Brown shared with my husband, Randy, and me his diagnosis of mild cognitive impairment (MCI). He had just received the diagnosis, and he said Randy was the first person other than his wife he had told. We have known Dave for many years, and we were stunned by the news. Dave had been reading about MCI on the Internet, and he had seen that, after five years, 50% of people diagnosed with MCI experience dementia. Randy recommended that Dave get a second opinion, which led him to receive exceptional care at the University of Washington's Harborview Medical Center in Seattle. At Harborview, they told him that his MCI was almost certainly the early stage of Alzheimer's disease.

Alzheimer's disease has no known cure, but Dave did substantial research on the disease and hit on a formula that seems to have effectively stopped the advance of the disease and reversed some of his symptoms. I have seen that what he has done has restored his confidence, self-esteem, and joy of life. His recommendations are worthy of being evaluated for incorporation into existing treatment regimens.

That said, let me share with you what I have observed in Dave over the past few years. I knew Dave as a friendly and self-assured man, but that began to change rather quickly after his diagnosis. He became confused and distracted, and he lost his confidence to a point where he decided to stop driving and resigned from his two jobs. He made responsible decisions, but his entire experience was emotionally devastating.

Dave wanted to do what he could to help himself. He actively sought help from his Harborview care team, evaluated their recommendations, and implemented them. He did a great deal of reading and examined the results of various clinical research studies. By trial and error, he established a regimen that worked for him. He began to notice a decrease in his depressive episodes, less inattentiveness, and improvement in his memory. His observations were validated by test results at Harborview and the VA hospital. The findings of the most recent test results indicate that the progression of MCI has stopped, and there was even some early evidence of reversal of the symptoms.

Of course, it is too early to know if his gains will be sustained over time, but what I do know is that he has regained his self-confidence and is driving again. Although he is not likely to return to work given his retirement age, he is more active and productive. He is volunteering at the Food Bank at least once a week, and he is participating in various activities involving his church and family. He says that the feeling of joy in life has returned. Outwardly, he seems more like the old Dave I knew before this started.

You may say that this all seems too good to be true. You may be right. But I know this: Dave's regimen has made a remarkable difference. What he recommends is practical, doable, and good for all aspects of your health, both physical and psychological. It is something that anyone confronting MCI should try to the extent that they are able. It could lead to gains in managing MCI that do not involve medical intervention.

When he began his treatment a few years ago, little did he know that he was finding a regimen that would be a key to success in helping him regaining the joy in his life. Dave is excited to share his findings with you, as I am. I hope you find his insights useful and make gains that will give you reason for joy.

Tae-Im Moon, Ph.D.,
Licensed Clinical Psychologist
November 2017
Richland, Washington

Introduction

I am not a doctor, I am not a research scientist, and I am not a journalist. I am one of millions of Americans who have been, or will be, diagnosed with Mild Cognitive Impairment, also called MCI. MCI is not in itself a disease, but it is a condition that likely signals the onset of one of several diseases. In my case, I'm told that it is likely Alzheimer's disease.

At the time of my diagnosis, I was 65 years old, in excellent health, gainfully employed in a job that I enjoyed, and looking forward to many more years of enjoying a productive life with a wonderful family. Suddenly, I found that it was not safe for me to drive a car, I was getting lost in conversations, I was making errors in my work that I had never made before, I was dizzy all of the time, and I was having regular episodes of a strange kind of depression.

I saw a neurologist who told me that I had MCI. I had never heard of MCI before. As I researched what my doctor told me, I became alarmed that I was a few short years from becoming so out of touch with the world that I would be a terrible burden on my family.

Over the past decade or so, I had developed a heart for the elderly. It was customary for me, after church on Sunday, to stop at two or three nursing homes and visit with friends suffering from dementia. I was fully aware of how dementia ravaged people's minds and of how rapidly it might advance.

While our recognition of my condition evolved over two or three years, it was 2015 when the whole load of bricks fell on us. I was evaluated at Harborview Medical Center in

Seattle where they administered a battery of psychometric tests and studied my brain with magnetic resonance imaging (MRI). The results were quite frightening.

It is now more than two years later, and I am driving daily and very safely. The dizziness is still present but much diminished. The depressive episodes, which once occurred three or four times per week, now occur in a very mild form less than once per month. I recently received cognitive test results that I would have been delighted with 20 years ago. It can still be a little harder for me to explain a complex idea, but these things are so much better than in 2015 and 2016. I also no longer have episodes where I sit on the sofa, staring out into space with no desire to speak with anyone.

I am not a medical or scientific authority on MCI and dementia. I cannot tell you authoritatively about the disease mechanisms, nor can I tell you authoritatively the state of dementia research with respect to beta amyloid plaques, tau proteins, and whatever else anyone thinks might be causing neurodegenerative diseases.

But I can tell you authoritatively about my own experience. I am an expert on that. I can tell you what I did, and I can tell you what my medical test results have been. I can tell you that I feel as though I have stepped back from the edge of a cliff.

I want to share my experiences because I believe that others can benefit. I doubt that everyone with MCI and dementia can benefit to the extent that I have because of my age and my otherwise good health. Central to my success has been getting to the gym and getting a vigorous workout every day. Some will not have the physical ability that I have, and they may experience less success. However, I do believe that what has worked for me is sure to help anyone at some level.

From what I read, I represent many, perhaps a million or more Americans between the ages of 60 and 75, who are experiencing MCI. Even if a fraction of these are the only ones who might benefit from following my strategy, many people might still be helped, and I'm sure there are many in their 70s and beyond who may benefit as well.

Because I am not an expert, you should not accept anything I say at face value. Do your own research, but rely on reliable resources. There are plenty of charlatans out there on the Internet pedaling questionable products and information based on half-baked theories. I always rely on genuine research conducted by legitimate scientists working in accredited institutions and following recognized scientific protocols. You should too.

How did I get here? What have I learned in the process? Is there help for others? I want to share my story, so here it is.

Chapter 1 – The Role of Traits in the Struggle

I WROTE THIS BOOK TO TELL THE story of how I have been able to deal with cognitive impairment and improve my life. My hope is that it will help others like me. The approach that I describe is somewhat dependent on personal traits, so it's best that I state up front what traits of mine I believe helped me to achieve the progress that I have. You can make up your own mind as to what extent you can safely apply my strategy to your own situation.

I received my diagnosis of mild cognitive impairment—MCI—when I was 65 years old. According to the Alzheimer's Association, there is very little statistical information available regarding the prevalence of MCI due to Alzheimer's disease in the United States. However, they say that 15% to 20% of Americans over the age of 75 have MCI. Additionally, 3% of Americans between the ages 65 and 74 have been diagnosed with full-blown Alzheimer's disease.[1] That's about

---

[1] Alzheimer's Association. "2017 Alzheimer's Disease Facts and Figures." *Alzheimer's & Dementia*. April 2017; Volume 13, Issue 4, Pages 325–373.

9 million of us. The people who will best benefit from my story are those who have been diagnosed with MCI and are in adequate physical condition to engage in reasonably vigorous aerobic exercise.

First, an important word of warning. My strategy depends very much on aerobic exercise, and I offer these cautionary stories:

> Our oldest son has a friend whose parents divorced when he was quite young. As a result, his father was estranged from his children for years, but he wanted to strengthen his bond with his son. He wanted to play sports with the boy, but he was not in good physical shape. Consequently, he joined a gym to lose weight and get into shape. At the gym, he climbed onto a treadmill and dropped dead from a heart attack.
>
> I also had a friend who went to the gym one day, got on a treadmill, and dropped dead from a heart attack. He was younger than I am now.

The moral of these stories is that if you are going to begin vigorous exercise after a sedentary period of your life, see your doctor first! As I will discuss later, if it's not safe to engage in vigorous exercise, or if you are otherwise unable to, there are alternatives.

My key traits

First, other than my MCI, I am in reasonably good physical condition. But this was not always so.

When I was in my 20s, I ran (and co? marathon race. Of course, I trained for the good physical condition at the time. But after variety of reasons, my level of physical fitness decin. steadily. When I was about 50, a middle school-aged son of mine said that I was "old, fat, and bald."

Weight and diet

I heard my son's challenge, and it got me thinking. I thought that I couldn't do anything about the old, and I wasn't likely to do anything radical about the bald, but I really should do something about the fat. I dieted to shed about 30 pounds. Over the years, those pounds have tried to come back, but I have kept them at bay.[2]

In the process of losing weight, one thing I learned was that diet will knock off pounds, but it takes a lot of exercise to make much of a weight difference—more than I'm willing to do. Therefore, I initially used SlimFast® to drop the pounds, and then I followed a low-carbohydrate approach in all of my eating to keep them off. I especially avoided the simple carbohydrates in corn sweeteners, refined sugar, and refined flour. I was inspired to follow the low-carb approach after reading *Dr. Atkins's New Diet Revolution*. While I have not recently been following Dr. Atkins's prescription with much rigor, the concepts in the book have guided my approach to

---

[2] I will discuss later how controlling simple carbohydrates and maintaining an appropriate weight can play a role in the evolution and control of some dementias.

ating for 15 years.   It is largely consistent with the Mediterranean diet that I now follow carefully.

The process of knocking carbohydrates out of my diet was difficult at first—the first two weeks were the hardest. But I noticed that, as time went on, my desire to eat carbohydrate-rich foods diminished. At one time, cheesecake and chocolate were my absolute favorite foods. However, after a period of time living without refined sugars and flour, neither cheesecake nor chocolate looked as appealing to me as they had in the past. I believe that once I shifted my metabolism away from carbohydrate-dependency, my mind shifted its focus to other, better sources of nutrition.

Controlling my weight this way has worked out reasonably well for me. Despite my 23andMe® DNA profile saying that I am genetically prone to be overweight, and despite controlling my intake of carbohydrates and calories being a daily struggle, I'm still able to stay close to my goal. As I write this, my height is 5' 6", and I weigh 148 pounds. That gives me a very favorable body mass index.

Personally speaking

You will read elsewhere that I am retired, at least for now. I felt forced into retirement by my MCI, but I may want to return to the workforce if things continue on their current path. I hold a baccalaureate degree in nuclear science from the State University of New York Maritime College, and I worked for many years as a nuclear engineer. I worked for 15 years as a civilian employee of the Navy, refueling and repairing submarines, and I worked about 20 years for the U.S. Department of Energy.

I have served in executive leadership roles in several organizations over the years. Some were religious, and others were secular.

In my early 50s, I attended night classes at Washington State University to receive a certificate to teach physics in Washington State high schools. For a decade, I went back and forth between substitute teaching high school and engineering consulting. I loved all of this.

Since my early college years, I have been fascinated by computers. In my 50s and 60s, I learned to apply several computer programming languages as a hobby. In my early 60s, I began to program Android apps in the Java computer language.

On my 59th birthday, the birthday fairy brought me a set of Rosetta Stone® discs for learning the Latin American brand of Spanish. With the help of the discs, the Internet, and a friend in Ecuador, I became fluent in Spanish—sufficiently so that I was able to teach biology in Spanish to immigrant high school students. This was during an eight-week period when the regular bilingual science teacher was out on maternity leave. Part of my Spanish learning process was to read the entire Bible in Spanish twice. While reading, I listened to a vocal narration to help with pronunciation.

This was a great experience, and I continue to practice my Spanish daily.

The role of faith in my life

I am a Christian, and my faith is a central feature of my life. It is, in fact, what guides me in my attitudes and decisions, and it contributed to my inspiration for writing this book. My morning routine includes more than an hour of quiet time spent reading the Bible and praying. I have read that these practices are beneficial to brain health, and I believe it.

I am a member of a conservative Lutheran denomination and a member of a small congregation where I served as executive director for about a decade.

Cognitive overhead

When I was evaluated for cognitive decline at Harborview Medical Center in Seattle, they assigned a rather high value to my pre-morbid IQ. They didn't have access to any pre-morbid IQ tests, so they inferred it from my education and professional experience. I certainly couldn't have scored well on an IQ test at the time they were evaluating me! Many years ago, however, I did score well on college entrance exams. In fact, I likely got into college on the strength of test scores, since I graduated somewhere near the bottom of my high school class.

So native intelligence has played a role in how the story of my life has unfolded, but I don't view native intelligence as a source of pride. It was something the Good Lord decided to give me at birth, and it conveys only responsibility. According to the Bible, "Everyone to whom much was given, of him much will be required, and from him to whom they entrusted much, they will demand the more."[3]

---

[3] Luke 12:48, ESV

Chapter 2 – Ominous Signs

SOMETIME IN 2011, I BECAME concerned about my balance and my ability to simply navigate our own home. When standing, I felt unsteady, and when turning the corner in the hallway, I would consistently bump my shoulder into the wall. What was going on?

Being unsteady

I remembered that my mother's father had a brain tumor, and I recalled that his symptom seemed to be the same as this.[4] Naturally, I began to wonder if I had a brain tumor.

The unsteadiness didn't go away, and I got a referral to a neurologist who had an MRI done of my head. The MRI didn't find the tumor I feared, but my problems persisted.

---

[4] The doctors concluded that a benign tumor the size of a golf ball behind his left eye was causing my grandfather's balance issues, and that's certainly logical. Nevertheless, he suffered from dementia in his 70s, and he complained to me about memory problems. While he blamed this on the surgery, I wonder now if perhaps his problems with dementia, balance, and memory were early indications of Alzheimer's instead.

The neurologist subsequently referred me for a number of tests of my vestibular system, but those also couldn't identify any problems.

The vestibular apparatus is located in the ear, and it passes information that the brain can use to understand the motion, balance, and orientation of the body. To the best of my recollection, the test lasted an hour or so, and they blew air into my ear. I don't know what they actually measured or how they measured it.

Losing joy

I recall from my 40s and 50s sitting in my office, sitting in a Bible study class, or just relaxing at home and thinking about how well I felt and how wonderful everything seemed to be. I would think about how satisfied I was with my professional achievements, how much joy my family gave me, and how positive I felt about dealing with every challenge.[5]

At the time I began experiencing balance problems I also had a sense that the joy was being drained from my life. One day, I was sitting in my urologist's exam room waiting for the doctor to come in. There was a poster on the wall listing a number of symptoms, one of which was a loss of joy. I read the list, and I said, "Hey, that's me." The poster advertised testosterone treatments.

When the doctor came in, I told him that I thought that I should get testosterone treatments because I was experiencing the symptoms on his poster.

---

[5] It is only in late 2017, after two years of fighting cognitive decline, that this sense of joy is returning in force.

"Absolutely not!" he said. "You don't want that!" He then went on to give me a long list of convincing reasons why I didn't want to mess with testosterone.

Keeping those balls in the air

For me, an early indication of my disease was a reduction in what I called "the number of balls I could keep in the air."

In my profession and civic activities, I've always been something of a workaholic. In addition to work responsibilities, several times I found myself at the helm of our church and other civic organizations. These activities were all time-consuming, and they also required thought to ensure the wheels would all turn as in a well-oiled machine. You can ask others about how successful I was at this, but I do know that I lived a stress-filled life—which I loved.

When people complained about stress or experts talked about reducing stress in your life, I chuckled. I told myself that I loved stress. I prided myself in how many balls I could keep in the air, all at one time. It was normal for me to be working on one thing or another all the way up until bed time. My main diversion was (and still is) photography, but I treated that as another job, requiring intense concentration for me to be successful at it.

One day, I realized that I just couldn't keep all of those balls in the air any more, and for the balls that I could keep up, I couldn't do those tasks as well as I could before. This became noticeable to others and embarrassing to me.

Time to worry

I became concerned about how well I was thinking. This was mostly at work where I was having trouble doing a good job reviewing complex documents. Especially if you are a knowledge worker, cognitive ability is the basis for your competence, and loss of cognitive ability will attack your self-worth.

In time, what had been unsteadiness became dizziness, and the dizziness contributed to a general sense of "un-wellness." I became very concerned about the problems with my balance, but I also began to worry how much longer I would be competent in my work.

I returned to the neurologist with a new complaint about cognition. He administered the "Mini-Mental State Examination" (MMSE) and concluded I had "mild cognitive impairment" (MCI).[6] This was January, 2015. During the test, I was stunned that after repeating a set of three words many times, I could recall only one of them after a few minutes. I had received a similar test a few years before to qualify for long-term care insurance, and I had easily remembered a set of about ten words after approximately 45 minutes.

As I understand it, MCI means that the brain is atrophying at a rate greater than with normal aging, and it can have many causes. However, I read that after five years, the majority of persons diagnosed with MCI suffer from full-

---

[6] I have since concluded that the MMSE is inadequate for a conclusive diagnosis of MCI, but its use in this way seems to be common.

blown dementia. When I first learned this, I became even more worried.

For reasons that became clearer later, the neurologist referred me for physical therapy for my balance. The physical therapist taught me a number of exercises that brought remarkable relief from the dizziness and the accompanying sense of un-wellness. These exercises continue to help me to this day.

The physical therapist also explained to me some things that the neurologist had not. He told me that the cause of my dizziness and sense of un-wellness was that the parts of my brain responsible for interpreting information from the vestibular system were dying. I was experiencing something like vertigo in the absence of a good sense of balance. The objective of the exercises was to have the brain re-learn functions that were lost with the dying cells. The therapist also mentioned several times that exercise would benefit me, but this wasn't part of his program. The idea that physical exercise would help my brain did not initially make a big impression on me.

The physical therapy began with a machine that I was to stand in. It was kind of a big box that gave me an artificial horizon and scenery. The entire box would tilt and roll, and I would need to remain standing as well as I could. There were other exercises in the clinic's gym where he would have me purposely become dizzy through head and body movements while walking.

When I had the gym exercises down, I stopped going for physical therapy. The clinic gym exercises were extremely effective, but I could do them at home. I still do them to this day when they are called for.

What I experienced

I believe that what I was experiencing is common to what others experience in MCI. We think of dementia in terms of memory loss, but, at least in Alzheimer's disease, the entire brain is dying. Caregivers, friends, and family of people with cognitive decline should understand what the sufferer is experiencing. My list is here:

- I felt unsteady. I needed to steady myself when standing, and I would sometimes hit my shoulder against the wall while rounding a corner in the hallway of our home. This was accompanied by a feeling of vertigo.
- I had frequent episodes of mild depression, often four or five times per week. These disappeared later in the evening and may have been what psychologists call "sundowning." They weren't overwhelming, but they were strong enough to take the fun out of life.
- I felt a little bit ill most of the time. This seems to have resulted from a combination of the vertigo and the mild depressions.
- I felt discouraged when I considered the loss I was experiencing. The loss of confidence in professional competence struck directly at my sense of self-worth as did the loss of confidence in my ability to drive safely.

- I was embarrassed to begin explaining a thought or an idea to someone and then become lost in the presentation.
- I began to have difficulty speaking. I sensed that my ability to control the formation of words in my mouth was eroding.

My struggle here has not been as bad as it has been for some others. I recall the expression of pain by someone at a support group meeting as he explained how frustrated and disappointed he was with himself when he was unable to do so many things he had in the past. His anger with himself and his loss of self-worth seemed to be eating him more than any of the other effects of his disease.

Chapter 3 – My Life Begins to Change

Each morning, I would drive to Starbuck's® on my way to work and pick up a dark Grande® coffee. Proceeding to work then required me to make a left turn after leaving the parking lot. One morning while making the turn, I slammed on the brakes because there was a pedestrian I hadn't seen crossing the street in the cross-walk. It occurred to me that the exact same thing happened in the exact same crosswalk after leaving Starbuck's a few days before. I realized that these had occurred because I had forgotten to look for pedestrians before making the turn. I had been turning left at this intersection for decades, but I had never done anything like this before.

Starbuck's wasn't the only place where I was experiencing this problem. Every now and then, my wife Amy and I would visit our children in Seattle about 200 miles away, and we would frequently go out in the evening to dinner together. I began noticing that I was having similar problems with pedestrians while driving to restaurants.

This was scary stuff, but the last straw occurred while I was driving out of town in broad daylight, and I nearly drove another car off the road. I was changing lanes when I heard a car honking, but I couldn't figure out what the honking was about. I looked in my side mirror and saw a car in the space I was trying to move into. I zipped back into my lane, and the other car went quickly on ahead.

This really shook me up. Though I managed to avoid causing an accident, I realized that I was not doing the simplest things necessary to drive safely, such as checking my mirrors before attempting a lane change. I was forgetting those skills. Worse yet, I was now struggling to make the mental connection between the sound of a car horn and how I was driving, a situation where timing is absolutely critical.

After this last incident, I immediately stopped driving and began walking to work. I relied on Amy to drive me to places I couldn't walk to.

Walking to work wasn't a bad idea anyway. According to my pedometer and Google Earth, it was a little more than a mile from our home to my office. Even during the winter, I found the walk was very pleasant and refreshing.

Frankly, I could also use the exercise. Some forty years earlier, I had completed a real marathon, but I had been rather sedentary since.

But, while walking to work, there was another hazard. I needed to cross a highway at a busy intersection. There were stop lights and pedestrian lights, but caution was still required to be safe. One day, I approached the intersection and waited for the light to change. While watching, I suddenly realized that I couldn't predict what the cars would do—which would turn and which would continue. It was only when I saw one car come up the road and turn right that

I realized that the cars traveled on the right-hand side of the road. Once I realized that, what all of the cars were doing made sense. I had known how traffic works all of my life, but I was now struggling to recall the most basic rules of the road.

To Harborview

But was this the end? I could walk to work, but I was less and less confident that I was doing a good job when I got there. The managers that I reported to thought I was doing fine and spoke well of me, but some of my co-workers weren't so sure. They probably had a better vantage than the managers. My neurologist hadn't offered any hope, but maybe there were other resources out there.

I spoke with a friend of ours who was a nurse. After checking with her associates, she said that I should go to the University of Washington Harborview Medical Center's Brain Wellness Center in Seattle. My neurologist gave me a referral to Harborview, and I was seen there. At Harborview, I was subjected to two days of testing that included physical testing (including for balance and walking), cognitive testing, and an MRI. This was June, 2015. After the testing, we went on a cruise to Alaska, and we returned afterwards to hear the results.

The diagnosis

When we returned to Harborview after our cruise, we met with the Harborview care team assigned to me, and they presented us with a grim outlook. The care team consisted of a neurologist, a neuropsychologist[7], a nurse practitioner, and a social worker. Their most significant observation was that my brain had atrophied noticeably between my local neurologist's initial MRI and the one conducted by Harborview. Without an autopsy(!), they couldn't present us with a definitive diagnosis, but they said that it was very likely Alzheimer's disease.[8] They could do some more brain scans to improve their confidence in the diagnosis, but the insurance company would never pay for it. Regardless of the results, my prognosis and treatment wouldn't have changed, so there was no point in further investigation.

An additional brain scan would have been positron emission tomography (PET). A PET scan can show how and where glucose is being metabolized in the brain, and Alzheimer's disrupts that metabolism. This is an important point that we will revisit later.

As we met with the care team, I was struggling somewhat to believe what was going on, and during our meeting, I minimized the day-to-day symptoms. This was probably denial. But my son, Darien, reminded us of an event a few weeks previously when I had found a watch on the table and thought it was his. When he told me that it was my own watch, I didn't believe him, despite the fact that it was the same watch that I had been wearing every day for 10 years.

---

[7] Neuropsychology is a subspecialty of psychology and requires additional training. Board certification in Clinical Neuropsychology shows competency in the subspecialty.

[8] I understand that a brain biopsy can be performed on a living person, but this is pretty radical and not warranted.

18

There were other examples of increasing problems with my memory as well.

I have learned a little of what they look for in MRIs. One thing they look at is the ventricles. The ventricles are fluid-filled void spaces in the brain that expand as the brain atrophies. Basically, the volume of the void space grows to compensate for the loss of brain tissue. They compared the size of the ventricles in my 2011 MRI to their own MRI, and they found that the ventricles were growing way too fast.[9]

They also measure hippocampus volume. I have read that the hippocampi (the two of them) play an important role in the consolidation of information from short-term memory to long-term memory and in spatial memory that enables navigation. I have also read that it is one of the first regions of the brain to suffer damage from Alzheimer's disease. My Harborview care team's analysis said that my hippocampus volume was in the 36 percentile for someone my age. In other words, 64 per cent of the population will have a larger hippocampus than mine. (In 2017, we would re-visit that and find that it may actually have been closer to the one percentile.)

As far as my psychometric (cognitive) test scores went, a quick look would say that maybe I did OK because a lot of them were assessed as "average." There about 35 individual tests, and more were "average" than any other result. While there were a few "Superior," more of the others

---

[9] It's natural for the aging brain to atrophy some, and for the ventricles to grow. However, atrophy accelerates significantly in Alzheimer's disease.

were "low average." However, the Harborview team said that, based on my education and professional achievements, I should have been rated "superior" on most of them. They said that I had a lot of "cognitive overhead"[10] (i.e., the Good Lord blessed me with a higher than average IQ at birth), and it was difficult to diagnose me simply on cognitive test results. They said that for my final diagnosis, they had to rely on my ugly MRI scan results.

Psychologists have a system for reconciling average, higher, and lower test performances with an individual's pre-morbid cognitive abilities. It's called the Montreal Cognitive Assessment©, and they scored me on this scale. They rated me "impaired."

It was shortly before this when I began to wonder if the mood swings—the episodes of mild depression—were part of the bigger picture of what was happening to me. I noted that these would usually occur four or five times per week. I also noted that they would start in the late afternoon and suddenly and dramatically disappear later in the evening. I had been reading and watching online videos about dementia, and I had come to believe that these were the "sundowning" I was hearing about.[11] Based on how the care

---

[10] Another term I have encountered is "cognitive reserve."

[11] According to what I've read, sundowning is attributable to the changing shadows in the later part of the day that can be upsetting to people with dementia. However, this pattern continued in the Alaskan summer, where changing shadows were minimal. I suspect the cause is deeper, and it is influenced by the circadian rhythm.

On the other hand, people who know more about this than I do tell me that a strong correlation has been established between

team quizzed me on this, I believe that they were coming to the same conclusion.

The care team recommended that Amy and I participate in a Mayo Clinic research study called "Healthy Action to Benefit Independence and Thinking," or HABIT®. They also gave us a list of life-style recommendations that included getting 20 minutes of exercise five days per week, reducing (but not eliminating) stress, and eating a Mediterranean diet with fish. They said, "What's good for the heart is good for the brain." They also added, "Don't quit your job."

I didn't immediately have 100% control of all of these, but I did my best to implement them. I learned to like salmon, and I reduced stress by quitting my job as executive director of my church. (This probably benefited the church as much as it did me.) My job wasn't terribly stressful, but our contract was slowly winding down, so the stress from work went down accordingly. I made some effort to up my game on exercise, but that was initially tentative.

---

changes in light and body chemistry associated with mood. It may be that my experience is not true sundowning.

Chapter 4 – Time to Get Serious

The HABIT® study

IN NOVEMBER 2015, AMY AND I STARTED with the HABIT study. We joined with a group of 11 other couples—participant and partner—for two weeks at a very pleasant senior living facility in Seattle. In most cases, a couple was a husband and wife, but in other cases, it was mother and offspring or participant and friend. We were told that the participants were all diagnosed with MCI, although it struck me that a few had declined significantly more than others. I could carry on a conversation with most of them, but two or three spoke haltingly. However, I never felt that anyone I spoke with would lose the thread of a conversation while I was speaking with them.

One of the first things I noticed about our group was that the participants were remarkable people who had achieved important things in their lives. One man had been a Washington State superior court judge who, after retirement, sailed the world with his wife. A couple of participants had been Christian missionaries in different countries around the world. The psychologist who conducted the support group sessions (and who was a principal investigator for the study) had been born in India, and one of the missionaries had his mission in the same village where she was born. I thought this was an interesting coincidence.

I also found that, at 66, I was the youngest person in the group.

The concept behind the study was to investigate five strategies for countering the progression and effects of our disease(s). The strategies would be tried in different groups across the country. The object of the study was to identify which areas of lifestyle during earlier stages of MCI might help to preserve participants' ability to maintain function as their disease progressed.

At the initial two-week session, we would begin with cognitive testing. The strategies then included making disciplined use of a calendar, playing computer games, support group sessions, yoga-based exercise, and education. (Of course, the yoga-based exercise was not aerobic.) Each group would omit one strategy. Our group omitted computer games, which I was glad about.

There were "booster sessions" at six month intervals over 18 months. Two of these meetings were one day meetings at the six-month and one-year marks. At the one-year meeting, the study researchers repeated the cognitive testing, but they didn't share the results with us. The results provided statistical data to support the study.

Support groups

I think that my favorite HABIT activity was the support group session. The participants were separated from their support partners, and the partners went to their own support group. In our group, we were given a workbook in which to record answers to different questions about our personal histories. Homework was to answer the questions at night and share our answers the following day. It appeared to me that about half of us actually did that; the rest of us winged it during the meetings.

We were to continue the books at home and bring them to the one-year booster session. I was the only one who did that. However, I also got the agreement of the administrators to apply a different strategy. I had started my autobiography a few years previously, but I wasn't making progress. I thought that finishing my autobiography would be an improvement over simply answering autobiographical questions in their book, and the administrators agreed that it was a good idea too. I eventually self-published my autobiography in 2017.

In the support group sessions, all of the participants seemed coherent, although some struggled to get their sentences out.

We are educated

I didn't especially enjoy the yoga sessions,[12] but the education modules were very good. One session in particular

---

[12] I don't want to sell the Yoga short. It's likely helpful to many people, but I followed my own program of meditation and exercise.

focused on diet and what studies had shown about diet and brain health. They emphasized the Mediterranean diet and the "DASH" diet. The DASH diet is the "Dietary Approach to Stop Hypertension." I will discuss diet in more detail later.

The facility served us a very nice lunch every day. However, the day after the education session on diet, I pointed out to the study administrators that the food we were served at lunch was a complete contradiction to what they taught us in the diet module. The next day, we had a very nice lunch based on the Mediterranean diet, but the day after that and for the rest of the term, it was back to the same old (non-brain healthful) stuff.

The education sessions did have a module on exercise, but I don't recall a strong emphasis on aerobic exercise of the type that I was beginning to engage in. However, it appeared to me that only about half of the participants were at an age or were in a condition of health where they could have attacked a program of vigorous aerobic exercise.

Writing it down

Another strategy was discipline in keeping a calendar. They gave us books for recording every commitment and every scheduled task or activity. Then there was a system for checking off completed items. Each couple met with a counselor at the end of the day to review how we were utilizing the system.

I did well with their paper calendar at the outset, but I had already been using the Google Calendar® on my phone and computer the same way. I had just been sloppy in how I applied the Google Calendar, and I had some missed commitments to show for it. I asked them if I couldn't just use my phone instead of their book but with heightened rigor. They agreed, but they gave me some conditions. I had to be able to assign priorities, and I needed to be able to check off tasks when they were completed. I could do all of that; I just needed to apply discipline.

And disciplined I was. I'm still effectively using the Google Calendar app to this day. The only problem is that Google "improved" the app a while ago in a way that made it more awkward to check off completed tasks.

I join the gym

Shortly after we returned from our initial two week-long HABIT meeting, I went down and joined a local gym.[13] It had just opened in a storefront a mile from our home, and it was perfect for my needs. The price was also right, especially with their old-people discount. I was enamored with their treadmills which were a significant improvement over the treadmill we had at home.

The treadmill in our home is one we've had for many years, and Amy still uses it regularly. However, it's a poor fit for me ergonomically, and it won't incline above 10°. Because of problems with my back, I have been unable to run for the past several years. If I hold on to the treadmill handles, I can walk at a clip of 4.3 mph, and I can get an additional, necessary result by inclining the machine to 15°. But if I ever raise the speed to even 4.4 mph, I have problems

---

[13] A shout-out to Club 24 Fitness, with locations in south central Washington and northeast Oregon.

with bursitis in my hip. The 4.3 mph on a 15° incline is therefore the best I can do, and it seems to be just right for the best outcome for my brain health. The treadmills at the new gym were perfect for accommodating my needs in this regard.

Keeping on keeping on

I have kept the exercise up. My daily routine is to rise at 5 or a little earlier in the morning and spend the first hour or so as my devotional time. I then have a cup of coffee and head straight to the gym. At the gym, I spend 45 minutes on the treadmill, and I do weight training on alternate days. That's 45 minutes of aerobic exercise every day, seven days per week, and weight training every second day.[14]

I had been following this routine when I tore my left rotator cuff. That hurt a lot, but it gave me an excuse to back off on the weight training. Based on what I'd read, most of the benefit for my brain was coming from the aerobic exercise anyway, so it didn't bother me to take a break from weight training. It was about seven months before I could go back to weights. While I did some lower body work during the seven months, it was not like that before the rotator cuff tear.

I should not sell weight training short. Muscle strengthening through resistance exercise helps prevent falls, which regularly cause serious injury to older people.

---

[14] I initially did 40 minutes per day with great success, but I raised it to 45 minutes in November 2017.

We have roots in Hawaii, so we go to visit family there at least once per year. To minimize lost exercise time, I always join a gym while I'm there, and I get to the gym there every morning to continue my program. None of the gyms has a 2-week plan, so I end up paying the initiation fee each trip and then paying for one full month. It's expensive, but it's very important to me.

Chapter 5 – Reading, Research, and Testing

AFTER BEING INTRODUCED TO the idea that I had MCI, I began reading about dementia and doing my own research. At first, I read that a cure for Alzheimer's disease is right around the corner, and something will be available for us in no more than two, maybe three years. But as I continued to read different articles, I began to conclude that this might not be the case. In fact, I learned that our understanding of the disease mechanisms was much less developed than I had thought, and the path to a drug intervention was very uncertain. In fact, it seems to have become even more uncertain in the time since I began my journey with MCI.

Of mice and men

As I continued reading, one thing kept showing up: exercise, diet, good sleep habits, stress management, and social engagement are our most powerful weapons in fighting dementia. Everything I read pointed to this, whether it was a news article about a study or a study report itself.

My brother-in-law watches television programming from Japan where an aging population is drawing attention to dementia. He shared with me some good documentaries on dealing with dementia. These always had the same message: get aerobic exercise and eat a Mediterranean diet. Make sure your Mediterranean diet has fish in it—no red meat.

I also read a lot about experiments with mice. As I understand it, some mice have been bred (or had their genes edited) to be prone to Alzheimer's disease for study purposes. In one study, three groups of mice were subjected to different conditions to promote or discourage exercise. In the first case, the mice ran on a wheel and got aerobic exercise. In the second case, they needed to climb a wall to get food. This simulated resistance (weight) training. In the third case, they were required to be sedentary.[15]

The result? The advance of Alzheimer's disease was significantly retarded in the mice that got aerobic exercise compared to the other two groups. Surprisingly, there was little difference between the sedentary mice and the mice that did their resistance training.

At the six-month HABIT booster session (May 2016), we met a new psychologist who was interested in my case. I had been making a concerted effort to get exercise and eat well throughout the period following our initial meeting, and I had begun to feel much better about how my mind was functioning. Not only did I feel sharper, but the mood swings had gone from several times per week to about once every

---

[15] I like to joke that they gave the mice a comfortable little couch and a tiny TV remote.

two weeks. I told him I was certain that exercise was helping me, and he said that was very likely the case.

How long before Alzheimer's kills you?

The psychologist said that he had just returned from a conference on dementia, and three papers had been presented on the effect of exercise on dementia. He said that all three papers had identified a strong effect, and it was important that I continue what I was doing. He drew a graph on some scratch paper showing my future—a declining line with a sharp drop-off to death at 75 years. Recall that Alzheimer's is a deadly disease that kills the entire brain, thereby killing the victim. He then drew another graph with a drop-off that did not occur until 85 years of age. He said the second graph showed what to expect if I simply keep up the exercise.

He said, "This is all we have to offer. There are no drugs and no other treatments that will stop Alzheimer's, so keep it up."

I told him that I read that exercise can actually regenerate brain cells. I had read in a news article that a hormone[16] is generated during aerobic exercise that promotes this, although I heard and read elsewhere that brain cells can't regenerate. Drawing a simple sketch on scratch paper, he explained that brain cells can be repaired

---

[16] As I will discuss later, the article was probably referring to the brain-derived neurotrophic factor protein, which is not actually a hormone.

and regenerated. He said that this happens during aerobic exercise.

Back to Harborview

In June 2016, we returned to Harborview for annual psychometric testing. The testing was conducted by the Harborview psychologist, but the results would be delivered a few weeks later during an appointment with my Harborview neurologist. We had a baseline in 2015, and I was anxious to see how things had changed. I had been exercising and eating right, and I felt much better than I had earlier.

When I say that I felt better, you should understand that I have rarely felt completely well since this all started in 2012. At least when standing, I usually experienced some level of unsteadiness, although the physical therapy exercises helped that a great deal. The unsteadiness seemed to cause vertigo or motion sickness, so there was often a small element of nausea with me. During 2015 and 2016, mood swings (likely sundowning) were a significant part of my life, and they detracted a great deal from my ability to enjoy life.

Alzheimer's kills the entire brain. Therefore, someone with Alzheimer's will experience problems in many areas of living besides memory problems. During 2015 and 2016, I would sometimes sit on the sofa, just staring into space. I would be uninterested in talking to anyone or doing anything. This behavior seemed unrelated to memory; it was a manifestation of my mood. The good news was that this behavior was receding.

As we departed from home to make our way to Seattle, I was very optimistic, hopeful for testing that would show that I was actually improving. I had now been exercising daily for about six months. Then a stop for gas quickly changed the mood.

When I was filling up at the gas station, I put my credit card in the machine, and it wanted to know my zip code. This is the same question the machine always asks when I use my card to fill up, and it shouldn't be hard to answer. After all, we've had the same zip code for 20 years. But that day, I couldn't remember what it was. I went around the car and asked Amy what it was, and she told me. The number she gave me worked, but it didn't sound familiar at all. The experience cast a shadow over my expectations for the rest of the trip.

After the testing, I felt very uncertain about what the results might say. I knew that I hadn't done badly, but I did feel that I had done more poorly than the year before. To receive the results, we scheduled a follow-up visit with my neurologist, and then we returned home.

About two weeks passed before we returned to Harborview, and I was quite anxious about what we would hear. When the neurologist came in, however, she was all smiles. She said she had great news—my year-over-year decline was in-line with normal aging. We had an upbeat conversation, and she gave me some papers with all of my test results. She told me about something they called "the practice effect." This means that the more you take their tests, the better you get at it, and your scores rise artificially.

Their assessment of my results considered the practice effect.

She also helped me with something I was hoping for—adding my name to a list of drug trials as possible participant. If something new and promising came along, I wanted to get in on the ground floor!

I took the test results home with me, and then I got the test results from 2015. I compared the 2016 results to the 2015 results and became discouraged again. It looked to me like my test scores were notably worse than the previous year. I could see that the change wasn't terrible, but if that was normal year-over-year decline, how does anyone make it to 75? And where was this "practice effect?" Understanding that the practice effect artificially raised the later score made it even harder to accept.

Reality check

In writing this book, I've gone back and reviewed my 2015 and 2016 scores again. Perhaps I was a bit emotional in my initial analysis of the results, since a clear decline is not now evident. Each of the 35 or so tests had a numeric raw score which was the basis for a conclusive "qualitative description." These could be "superior," "high average," "average," "low average," or "below average." Ten of the qualitative descriptions changed between 2015 and 2016. Five had gone down, but five had gone up.

Another problem is that I don't know what I'm doing when I review these results. I'm not a psychologist, and I'm guessing at the significance of what I'm reading. I certainly don't know how to weigh the impact of the practice effect and other considerations on the scores and results.

Assessing where I'm at

Looking out at my future, I was still working, but the two contracts I was working on were winding down. I would essentially be out of work by December. This wasn't going to be a financial issue, but it went against the advice they'd given me: "Don't quit your job." In the past, I had one or two brief periods of unemployment, and these had been emotionally difficult. I wondered if being suddenly retired like this would have similar effects that would aggravate my MCI.

The 2016 testing reflected the results of six months of daily exercise. Regardless of what they told me, I concluded that six months of daily exercise had slowed, but not stopped, the progress of the disease. Maybe exercising seven days per week for a whole year would give me better results in 2017.

Chapter 6 – Being a Guinea Pig

AFTER PLACING MY NAME ON a list of study volunteers in 2016, I began to get calls. The first call was for the third stage trial for a drug that was supposed to clean out amyloid plaques.[17] The trial would be conducted in Seattle, and I needed to go there for screening. The name of the drug was Aducanumab. Say that three times fast.

Aducanumab

We had some reservations about the trial. Safety with any drug is important, and it is even more so with a new drug. This was a third-stage trial, and the first two trials had shown problems with "micro-hemorrhaging" in some brains. The trial would involve monthly visits to Seattle, sometimes twice in a month. Some visits would include MRIs to check for hemorrhaging and other physiological problems the drug might cause. For us, getting across the Cascade Mountains in the winter can be dicey, and we thought hard about making a commitment to be in Seattle on specific dates.

---

[17] I discuss the role of amyloid plaques in Alzheimer's disease and how Aducanumab removes them in the appendix.

The drug's history was troubling to us in other ways. Results from the first trial were positive, and they stirred a lot of interest. The stock price of the sponsoring drug company had jumped nicely when the results were reported. As I understand it, however, first-stage trials are mostly focused on safety, and they use a small population of subjects. It's likely that the seemingly positive results on the first trial were statistical anomalies, since the larger second-stage trial showed very little improvement among the subjects. That probably drove the company's stock price down. My question then was, why are they going ahead with the third-stage trial when the second stage showed the drug was probably not effective?

As a matter of coincidence, we met a researcher who happened to be in Seattle at the same time we were. He was knowledgeable of the drug, and he was skeptical of the concept behind its operation. A component of Alzheimer's theory was that the buildup of amyloid plaques on brain cells inhibited the flow of information from cell to cell. Therefore, if you remove the plaques, you speed up the flow of information, and the effects of Alzheimer's are controlled. Some also believe that the plaques kill brain cells. If that's correct, deposition of amyloids is a main feature of the disease process.

The researcher instead said he believed that the amyloids were simply an inconsequential byproduct of the disease process. It's useful for showing someone has Alzheimer's disease, but he believed that controlling amyloids controls neither the disease nor its negative consequences.

40

Washed out. Then what?

I did go through with cognitive testing for eligibility for the Aducanumab trial, but I failed the test. I scored too well, and my decline was considered insufficient to qualify me as a good trial subject. I attribute this to the effect of the diet and exercise because I'm sure I'd have performed much more poorly in 2015. On the other hand, my native cognitive reserve was also likely a factor.

The woman who administered the test then told me about another drug trial being run at the VA hospital in Seattle. She put me in touch with the coordinator, who told me that I was likely a good candidate. He sent me material that I would need for enrollment, and I was quite enthusiastic about participation. But later, he called to tell me that the sponsor had closed the door to new test subjects. They were all full. What a disappointment!

However, he said that he had another trial coming up where he felt confident that I could get in. I had him send me the details.

Insulin—a new possibility

It turned out that this was not a drug trial with a new drug but rather a novel use of insulin. The concept was that the brain is one of the biggest users of glucose in the body, and therefore it needs a lot of insulin. This is why the PET scan is a valuable tool in studying Alzheimer's disease—it shows how and where in the brain glucose is being metabolized. It detects breakdowns in the processes by which glucose is used in the brain.

Since Alzheimer's disrupts the processes in the brain by which glucose is acquired by cells and metabolized, increasing the concentration of insulin in the brain should improve brain function. Is that true? There is only one way to find out—raise the concentration of insulin in the brain and see what happens. But raising the concentration of insulin in the bloodstream to the levels they were thinking might be necessary would cause the whole body to be hypoglycemic, an undesirable condition. How do you raise the concentration in the brain without raising it in the rest of the body?

I suppose that the cocaine users know the answer to that one—snort it. If insulin could be blown into the nose, perhaps it could find the same path to the brain as cocaine.

As I understand it, at the top of the nasal cavity is a patch of tissue through which the olfactory nerve passes, and it is quite permeable to different substances. This pathway then bypasses the blood-brain barrier and permits some substances to enter the brain in high concentrations. The concentration of insulin in the brain might then be raised without raising it in the rest of the body. Apparently, someone thought the idea was sufficiently worthy to fund it.

I volunteered for the trial, and I went through the screening process. The screening process included an MRI, which I will discuss later. The MRI showed that my hippocampus volume was now in the ominous one percentile, but I was still concerned that I would not be admitted to the trial because of good cognitive test results. As I understand it from talking with the study coordinator, this almost turned out to be what happened. However, they did find enough justification outside of the cognitive tests to justify my admission to the drug trial. As of this writing, I am still participating.

Living with insulin

So how did the insulin trial work? The trial runs 18 months, and as I write this, I'm nine months into it. One half of the participants is receiving actual insulin, and the other half is receiving a placebo. At the 12-month mark, we will each be asked whether we believe we are receiving insulin or the placebo. The trial will then go "open label," and all participants will be using insulin. The placebo will be removed, and the trial will continue for another six months.

A second MRI will be administered at 12 months, and there are checkups quarterly. At initiation,[18] six months, 12 months, and 18 months, they perform thorough physical and cognitive examinations. At three months, nine months, and 15 months, the checkups involve a minor physical exam and some less extensive cognitive testing. I'm told that, following completion of the whole trial, I will be able to continue with use of the insulin at no cost until it is approved for clinical use.

How is the insulin administered? The investigators have designed a device that looks like an inhaler, the sort that might be used by someone with asthma. But instead of the asthma inhaler's large conduit that goes into the patient's

---

[18] I thought my initial physical examination was one of the most thorough I had ever received.

mouth, there is a smaller tube angled in the upward direction. The user loads small tips with insulin and mounts them on the tube. Then, as with an inhaler, pushing down on the propellant canister will atomize the insulin, and the spray can be directed into the patient's nose. The angle of the tube is such that the spray will impinge on the tissue at the top of the nasal cavity. From there, it can be absorbed and travel to the brain.

I perform this procedure twice per day. As I understand it, I am administering the insulin at the times when the glucose concentration in the blood should be at a peak. This is about one half hour after breakfast and one half hour after supper.

In May 2016, Amy and I returned to the VA hospital in Seattle for the three-month checkup required by the insulin trial protocol. The testing was similar to the cognitive testing they conducted at the outset of the trial, but it was less intense, and it did not take as long to perform. They did not share the results with us, but I felt that I did well enough. I had taken quite a few of these tests now, and I could tell that my performance was improving. (No doubt, the practice effect was helping with this.)

A favorite test method is to have the participant subtract seven from some number. The participant is then asked to subtract seven from that result, and then subtract seven from that result. In my initial MMSE in 2015, the neurologist started with 100, and I know that I blew it badly. (This should have been 100-7=93, 93-7=86, 86-7=79, etc.) The same occurred in my first testing at Harborview in Seattle,

except that they started with 109. I blew
With each test, however, I can't help b
question, and I am now better prep∂
regardless of the starting number.

So this is how the practice effect works. Whenever ι .
well about how I did on a test I come back to this and wonder
how it might be skewing my results.

Stunning results

I returned to the VA hospital for periodic testing in
August and November 2017. They did not share the results
of cognitive testing with me for either visit, but I felt well
about both sets of tests. In fact, I felt extremely well about
my performance on the November test set.

In November, I was shown 10 cards with words on them.
I read each card out loud in turn, and I was then asked to
recall the words on as many cards as I could. I didn't get
them all, but I believe I got most of them correct. The test
. then required me to read each card again and then recall all
that I could. On the second run, I recalled nine of the 10
cards correctly.

I was then told to read one time through the words in
another stack of 10 cards. The cards were turned over, and I
read each word out loud. I did this only once. Next, the
person administering the test turned over cards from a
second stack of about 20 or 25 cards, one at a time. (I didn't
count the cards; I'm only estimating.) This last stack
contained all of the words in the previous stack but many
others as well. As each card was turned over, my task was to
state whether the word on the card was or was not one of the

words in the previous stack. For every single card, I orrectly stated whether or not the word was or was not in the stack of 10.

This was a dramatic change from the test my local neurologist administered in 2015. At that time, I could only recall one of three words after he drilled me repeatedly on the three words.

Chapter 7 – Going Forward

A M I HOLDING MY OWN, have I slowed my decline, or am I actually getting better? I feel better, but what are the objective measures that can inform me? And what am I doing today that seems to be working?

Placebo uncertainty

Am I receiving true insulin or a placebo? Does it even work? If it does work, is it creating in my brain a dependence on an artificial insulin supply? Are there long-term ramifications, regardless of whether or not the insulin improves cognition?

I suspect that I have the placebo, but I'm not sure. I had been improving steadily prior to beginning the trial, and subsequent improvement seems to be an extension of the improvement process that was already in motion. After nine months, I feel that I've improved (and my cognitive test results support this), but has insulin actually brought something new, or is this simply the result of persistence at the gym continuing to pay off?

Cognitive testing

First and foremost are my test scores. These are the most objective measure of improvement. Sensations and mood are also important, but they are harder to quantify.

I became serious about exercise half-way between my Harborview tests of June 2015 and June 2016. You will recall that they told me that the year-over-year decline in my scores between 2015 and 2016 was in line with normal aging, but when I compared the scores myself, it looked to me (incorrectly) that my later scores were too much lower than 2015 to be attributable solely to normal aging. Also, it was while traveling to Seattle to receive the 2016 Harborview tests that I couldn't remember our zip code of 20 years. Soon after the episode with our zip code, I had an episode in which I couldn't remember our phone number. However, nothing like this has recurred.

While I found my 2016 results discouraging, 2017 was a different matter. I felt very confident following the testing, and my read of the results was that there was no decline at all. Of the 35 tests, 13 had changed from 2016. Five had gone down, but eight were higher. I don't recall exactly how the neurologist characterized the results—the test results spoke for themselves. She did say that she was very happy with them. So were we.

The results showed that progress of the disease has certainly stopped, and my November 2017 test results provide objective evidence of actual reversal.[19] The insulin study test results have been very encouraging, but their protocol requires that they not share the results with me. Nevertheless, it's hard to overlook the differences between how I was able to answer their test questions in February and November. Even more so, it's hard to overlook the differences from early 2015. I look forward to my next MRI in the hope that it will show physiological improvement.

Scanning the brain

My Harborview care team had said that they couldn't rely on cognitive testing for my initial diagnosis because my native cognitive abilities were well above average. My scores were in a very normal range, but they knew I should have scored significantly higher. They said that they instead relied primarily on the MRI results to conclude I had MCI. They found that the ventricles had grown, and my hippocampus volume had shrunk.

I have come to believe that MRI interpretations can vary depending on the MRI machine used, the software used to interpret the results, and the radiologist who interprets the results. Both of the 2017 MRIs reported similar results, but

---

[19] While writing this book, I compared my raw numerical scores from 2017 with my raw scores from 2015. I noted that 17 of the 2017 scores were higher than 2015. This was out of about 35 individual scores. But, for several reasons, this analysis is not very meaningful. Most importantly, many of the scores were only marginally higher and almost certainly lacked statistical significance. Nevertheless, this gives me great encouragement!

they showed that my hippocampus volume could now be measured such that I was in the one percentile.

Atrophy of the hippocampus is important. As I discussed earlier, the hippocampus plays an important role in processing short-term memory. According to articles I've read, its atrophy can be an early marker for the onset of Alzheimer's.

Harborview does not plan another MRI, and our insurance company would likely not pay for one if they did. However, the insulin trial protocol requires another MRI at the 12 month mark, and I anticipate that my Harborview neurologist will be able to review its results with me. I am hopeful that it will show improvement in my hippocampus volume. As I will discuss later, research has shown that aerobic exercise in older adults has been correlated with hippocampus volume *increases* of as much as 2%.

Balance

My adventure began when I experienced problems with balance. My neurologist originally suspected problems with my vestibular system,[20] but testing failed to confirm this. When it became clear that my problem could be related to the early stages of Alzheimer's disease, my physical therapist taught me exercises that I could do to combat balance problems.

---

[20] You can use Google to learn about the physiology of the vestibular system, but it is located in the ears. It provides information to the brain that is used to maintain balance.

The exercises included an activity in which I stand on one foot, or I stand with two feet aligned one behind the other, such that my balance is challenged. Then I move my head back and forth as well as up and down to further challenge my balance. (I do this standing by the kitchen sink so I can catch myself if I begin to fall.)

Another activity is to pace between two points about 30 feet apart while moving my head in circles. This induces dizziness, but I continue pacing. (I have never fallen while doing this exercise, but I am careful to walk a path that avoids dangerous places to fall.)

These exercises accomplish the re-training of my brain that my physical therapist told me about. The re-training compensates for the brain cells lost to Alzheimer's. I haven't been able to confirm his explanation, but neither have I seen anything to contradict it.

These exercises are remarkably effective. If I neglect them, I experience vertigo, and I can become nauseated. If I spend 10 minutes on them, I will be free of symptoms for several days, although it may take a day or so after the exercises to produce their full benefit.

I get a similar effect from the treadmill. When on the treadmill, I hang on to help maintain a rapid pace without actually running. (I have problems with my back and hip if I actually run.) While I'm doing this, I close my eyes and move my head around. I move it back and forth as well as up and down. This seems to be almost as effective as the exercises that the physical therapist taught me.

The fact that the condition returns after a few days tells me that the disease process is continuing, at least in the parts of the brain that are associated with balance.[21]

My lifeline—the treadmill

I now believe that my life absolutely depends on the treadmill. I believe that daily aerobic exercise, more than any other factor, has turned my condition around, at least for the foreseeable future.

An article in the *Proceedings of the National Academy of Sciences* described research[22] that correlated aerobic exercise to changes in hippocampus volume. The article concluded that aerobic exercise was effective in reversing hippocampus volume loss with attendant improved memory function.[23] To me, the key words here are "reversing" and "improved." I'm hopeful that this is not just about stopping progress of the disease but reversing the damage.

How does this work? My initial reaction was that improved blood flow to the brain must be helping, and other people I meet jump at that explanation as well. However, I've read elsewhere that exercise promotes the production of a

---

[21] These parts are likely the brain stem and the cortex. From what I read, they do not include the hippocampus. I understand that it's neurogenesis—regeneration of brain cells—in the hippocampus that is most affected by aerobic exercise.

[22] Erickson, Kirk I. et al. "Exercise training increases size of hippocampus and improves memory," *Proceedings of the National Academy of Sciences of the United States of America.* Vol. 108, no. 97, February 15, 2011.

[23] Erickson reported hippocampus volume increases of as much as 2%.

protein that participates in the "neurogenesis" process that repairs and regenerates the brain cells. The protein is called "brain-derived neurotrophic factor," or BDNF.

Staying connected to the human race

Two of the recommendations Harborview gave me at my initial diagnosis were "reduce but don't eliminate stress" and "don't quit your job." I was able to reduce stress by passing the baton for my role as executive director of our church. While it's a wonderful congregation, and I felt I had made a contribution, it really was time (maybe past time) for someone else to take over. That transition went a long way, and the church is doing just fine with someone else in that role.

"Don't quit your job" was a different matter. The company I worked for had me on two projects. One project was local and required that I go into the office every day. The other was more than 2,000 miles away in Tennessee, and I worked alone at home. Working at home provided very little human interaction. The local project was actually winding down as the company completed its mission, and I didn't see a future for me with the project in Tennessee.

After some discussion with my boss, I effectively retired in December 2016. As it is, my name is still on the books, and if the right task comes along, I could still go back to work. For now, however, I'm at home writing.

But why did they say, "Don't quit your job?" As I discussed elsewhere, some researchers say that something really important happens in social connection. I sense this because there were times in 2015 and 2016 when I was struggling with my cognitive function, and I also felt an urge to withdraw. This was when I would sit on the sofa with no desire to speak with anyone. Social engagement required me to push past a barrier, perhaps re-training the brain in some social skill.

Therefore, I do my best to maintain ample social connection. First, I went down to the food bank and signed up as a volunteer. This is really cool because I get to ride around in trucks with other old guys, stopping to pick up donations from different supermarkets.

I also continue to teach three Bible study classes per week. I have a small class of older adults on Sunday mornings, a class for elderly people in a retirement home on Tuesday mornings, and a larger class of mostly Millennials on Wednesday evenings. We begin the Wednesday class with a pizza dinner, and we enjoy social time together.

I love photography, and a friend had me join a local photography club. Monthly meetings and outdoor photo shoots provide more social activity.

This is how I stay engaged, and I believe that this also contributes to how well I've been doing.

What to eat

I will discuss different diets in more detail later, including how diet may (or may not) be helping me. I have adopted the Mediterranean diet, modified somewhat along the lines of the MIND diet. I eat blueberries, strawberries, walnuts, spinach, broccoli, tomatoes, wild Alaska salmon, avocado (have you seen the prices lately?), almonds, olive oil, eggs, and some poultry.

I also struggle controlling my weight, but I've been pretty successful keeping it down by following the low-carbohydrate regimen of these diets. It helps that the longer I'm on a low-carb diet, the less appealing high-carb foods are to me. It was an easy transition to a Mediterranean diet because of similarities between the low-carb and Mediterranean diets.

Losing your voice

Early in my experience, I noticed that I was having increasing difficulty forming words with my mouth. This was most noticeable—and problematic—when I was trying to teach a class. When I reported this to my Harborview care team, they asked me if I wanted speech therapy. I declined because I didn't think it was warranted. But my sense at the time was that my report didn't surprise them. I inferred from this that speech problems may be a characteristic of Alzheimer's disease. I looked into the question and found articles indicating that speech problems often appear in stages of the disease later than MCI.

Following my 2017 annual evaluation at Harborview, I enrolled in a study to follow changes in the speech of elderly patients. I now submit a voice sample to the research team monthly, and a computer evaluates them for changes and trends. The study correlates changes in speech with the advance of a variety of diseases, including Alzheimer's, Parkinson's syndrome, and ALS—Lou Gehrig's disease. The hope is that computer analyses will be able to identify characteristic voice changes associated with them. From this, they may be able to develop a diagnostic tool for early identification of emerging neurological disease.

Timeline of my Adventure

2012	2013-2014	2015	2016	2017	2018
• 3/12 - MRI for balance problems. No issues. MRI is baseline for future MRIs.	• Balance and dizziness grow steadily worse. • Begin to worry about cognition.	• 1/28 - Local neurologist diagnoses MCI based on MMSE. • 5/14-15 - Evaluation at Harborview w/MRI. MCI diagnosis confirmed. MRI shows hippocampus atrophy (36 percentile) and ventricles enlarged. • Late summer – stop driving due to near-misses. Start walking to work. • 10/26-11/6 – HABIT study begins in Seattle. • 12/15 – Join a local gym and begin daily treadmill exercises.	• Late spring – slowly returning to driving. • 6/13 – Annual psychometric testing/ evaluation at Harborview. Decline from 2015 in line with normal aging. • Summer – on the trip to Seattle can't recall zip code. A month or so later can't recall phone number. • Fall and winter – feeling much better. Daily aerobic exercise continues. Cognition clearly improving, mood swings much less frequent, driving is unimpaired. • 9/13 – Rejected from first drug trial due to high cognitive test results.	• 1/30, 2/13 – Two MRIs at UW. Both show ventricles unchanged from 2015. • 2/27 – Begin insulin study. • 6/21 – Annual psychometric testing/ evaluation at Harborview. No decline from 2015. • 5/31, 8/28 – Insulin study tests. Results not shared, but my sense is that I did well. • Sept – Begin participation in voice study. • 11/27 – Remarkable performance on cognitive test for the insulin study	• February - First phase of insulin study to end. MRI for comparison to Feb 2017 MRI. Will learn who had placebo. Study will continue 6 more months with no placebo. • June – Annual psychometric testing/ evaluation at Harborview. What will it show? • August – Insulin study to end. If effective, will continue with insulin pending government approval. • Voice study to continue.

Chapter 8 – The Remedies

IN THIS CHAPTER, I WANT TO provide my take on the different strategies that I understand people apply to prevent or treat Alzheimer's disease. I will begin with the strategies that I've applied successfully, but I will also try to touch on some others. To the best of my ability, I will sort them in the order of what I believe to be most to least beneficial.

Again, I am not an expert. What I write about here is from my personal experience, from what knowledgeable people have told me, and from what I've read.

First and foremost: aerobic exercise

If you haven't figured it out already, I believe that aerobic exercise is the single biggest factor in my improved cognition. If you are serious about dealing with cognitive decline, and you are otherwise healthy enough, you should begin a program of regular aerobic exercise, and you should do it soon. (**But please remember my caution at the beginning of chapter 1.**)

I discussed earlier why scientists believe aerobic exercise can be so valuable. It is because during aerobic exercise, the body produces the protein called brain-derived neurotrophic factor—BDNF. BDNF repairs damaged brain cells and participates in the generation of new brain cells, especially in the vitally important hippocampus part of the brain.

Diet and other factors contributing to our brain health get a lot of attention in science and the media. However, scientists are beginning to wonder if they have adequately controlled their studies for exercise. People with one healthful habit tend to adopt the whole suite of healthful habits. People who eat well also tend to be people who get exercise. Therefore, if research suggests that a good diet correlates with a lower incidence of Alzheimer's, is that because the diet is effective, or is it because the people who follow good diets also get a lot of exercise? This question is getting new attention from researchers.

How much exercise is enough? Any exercise is better than nothing! Even if the most you can do is just walk around the block, do it.

When I was given my diagnosis, I was told that I should get 20 minutes of aerobic exercise, five days per week, but is that enough to actually stop the disease? I've read other recommendations from researchers that recommend 45 minutes to an hour, six days per week. I've also read that organizations making recommendations have been known to understate what may be required for fear of scaring people away. On the other hand, I've heard some prominent researchers say that, beyond 30 minutes per day, five days per week, they believe there are diminishing returns.

I've read that good aerobic exercise will produce sweat after 10 minutes of work at room temperature. Also during good aerobic exercise, it should be difficult to speak in complete sentences, and your heart rate should reach 65% of maximum for your age. Google can help you find your maximum heart rate, but I think it's enough to make sure that you sweat on time.

I understand not wanting to scare people away, and I'm certain that even a small amount of exercise will help some. However, if you want to seriously slow, stop, or reverse the progress of the disease as I have, you will need to be more aggressive.

I have been getting 40 to 45 minutes of aerobic exercise per day, seven days per week for two years, and I have missed very few days. (These were usually days committed to air travel.) I am very satisfied with the results, and my recommendation is that, if you can, you should do the same.

What about weight training? Weight training has its benefits, but what I've read suggests that it does not help significantly with cognitive decline. As I mentioned before, it can still be very important for older people who are subject to falls. Additional body strength steadies people as they walk and can be valuable when a falling person must catch themselves.

Every little bit helps

Kristine Yaffe at UC San Francisco is a rock star in dementia research. In 2001, she and her team published a study which correlated the degree of cognitive decline with the distance older women walked and how much stair-climbing they did on a regular basis.[24] This was what researchers call a "longitudinal study" in which they followed the same women (nearly 6,000) over a period of six to eight years. These were predominantly white women aged 65 years and older who, at the outset, did not live in institutions and displayed no evidence of cognitive decline.

The research considered how many blocks the women walked per week, how much they climbed stairs, and how much energy they expended. The study controlled for age, educational level, the presence of other diseases, smoking status, estrogen use, and functional limitation. Cognitive status was measured by repeating a modified Mini-Mental State Examination.

So what did they find? The results were remarkable.

The women were divided into quartiles based on how much they walked each week. Women in the first quartile walked 0-22 blocks per week, women in the second quartile walked 23-49 blocks per week, women in the third quartile walked 50-112 blocks per week, and women in the fourth quartile walked 113-672 blocks per week. The median was 49 blocks per week, but 10% didn't walk at all and got no

[24] Yaffe, K. et al. "A prospective study of physical activity and cognitive decline in elderly women: women who walk." *Archives of Internal Medicine*. 2001 Jul 23;161(14):1703-8.

other regular exercise. The latter were obviously in the first quartile.

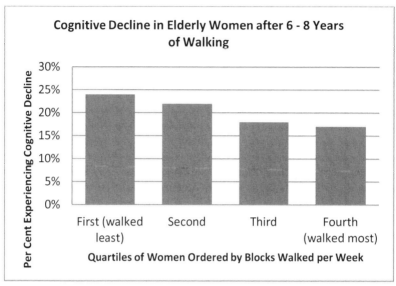

Figure 8-1 – Study results correlate walking among older women with a decrease in cognitive impairment. The women were divided into four "quartiles" containing equal numbers of women. The women in the first quartile walked the least and experienced the most decline, and women in the fourth quartile walked the most and suffered the least decline. (Yaffe et al., 2001)

As you can see from the graph, the women who made up the one quarter of the women who walked the most each week (the fourth quartile as I have displayed it) were the least likely to experience measurable decline. The women in the first quartile walked the least and were the most likely to experience decline.

The conclusion stated, "Women with higher levels of baseline physical activity were less likely to develop cognitive decline. This association was not explained by differences in baseline function or health status. This finding supports the hypothesis that physical activity prevents cognitive decline in older, community-dwelling women."

Being sociable

People with Alzheimer's withdraw socially, and I think we've come to accept that. We might assume that people with Alzheimer's want to withdraw because they're embarrassed about their disease or because they're depressed over their prospects.

It was during the year following my diagnosis that I sometimes found myself sitting on the sofa and staring into space. When I thought about talking with someone else, I was repelled by the idea. There are some researchers who believe that fighting the desire to withdraw socially also fights the advance of the disease.

I spoke with one researcher who had a neurology practice of 20 years. We talked about exercise, and he said that, in his experience, people who go to the gym by themselves go downhill just as fast as people who don't get exercise. He said that people who get exercise in a social setting don't decline nearly as rapidly. His example was people who go bicycle riding with friends. I would think that people playing golf with friends would also benefit.

I do have to disagree somewhat with what he said. While I go to the gym by myself and only rarely socialize there, I do stay active in my church, and I do volunteer work at the food bank. My situation began to change when I upped my game on exercise, not when I started socializing more. (I didn't.) I believe that both my new exercise regimen and continuing social activity are doing their parts. However, I am certain that exercise is the most important.

How important is diet?

People go quickly to the diet question. We all know that you are what you eat, so the nutrients and other chemicals going into our bodies will influence many aspects of our health. It's a natural assumption that eating the wrong things might cause Alzheimer's, and eating the right things might remedy Alzheimer's. Surely, there are things you may be eating that will hurt many aspects of your health, including brain health.

As I read more on this topic, however, I'm increasingly skeptical of the central importance of diet. I mentioned before that people who eat well also tend to get more exercise, and that likely explains much of the statistical correlation between diet and cognitive decline. I discuss elsewhere that obesity and diabetes are important risk factors for Alzheimer's, and diet is important in controlling these. Consequently, people exercising regularly and controlling their weight through a good diet will be less vulnerable to Alzheimer's.

That being said, we should not miss any opportunity to improve brain health. Even if, for many of us, the influence of diet might be overshadowed by exercise, I still follow dietary recommendations from sources that I trust. This is especially true where eating a recommended diet is not much different from what I was eating anyway.

Neurologists are fond of saying, "What's good for the heart is good for the brain." This certainly applies to exercise and to diet, so the brain-healthy diets begin as heart-healthy diets.

About carbohydrates

Another thing researchers state repeatedly is that keeping consumption of carbohydrates low is fundamental to brain health. I have learned to examine the nutritional information on the labels of every food I eat, and I look to see what the "net carbs" are for what I'm about to consume.

Net carbs are the total carbohydrates, minus the dietary fiber. For example, if you read on the label that a single serving has 25 grams of total carbohydrates and 5 grams of dietary fiber, your net carbs will be 20 grams.

Why is this so? Dietary fiber is largely cellulose, which is a form of glucose that is not digested by humans. (It's a different story for goats.) Since cellulose is a carbohydrate, it counts as total carbohydrates, but it is not a factor in weight control and brain health.

Some approaches to carbohydrate control recommend maintaining your intake below 100-150 grams per day while others have been as low as 20-50 grams per day. This is difficult, and it requires some discipline to maintain these levels. Nevertheless, after you have trained your body to accept a low level of carbohydrate intake, my experience is that the high-carb foods begin to look less appetizing.

This discipline will lead you to avoid some high-carbohydrate foods traditionally thought to be healthful. For example, I don't eat rice, potatoes, bananas, or oranges. I can get the same benefits from broccoli, blueberries, strawberries, avocados, and other healthful foods with lower net carbohydrate content.

Why is it important to control carbohydrate intake? High levels of carbohydrates in the blood contribute to the evolution of "insulin resistance" in the brain. Glucose is the brain's only source of energy, and it uses a lot of it. Insulin "signals" cells to take up and use glucose from the blood stream, but resistant cells do not properly accept the signal from insulin, and they become starved for glucose. As insulin resistance advances, we call it type 2 diabetes.[25] A three-hour fast between dinner and bedtime and a twelve hour fast from dinner to breakfast give the cells a rest. This fights insulin resistance and helps against type 2 diabetes. Aerobic exercise is another significant factor in the prevention of insulin resistance.

Disruption of the metabolism of glucose in the brain is a feature of Alzheimer's disease.[26] Therefore, insulin resistance and diabetes are recognized risk factors for Alzheimer's disease. (Obesity is also a recognized risk factor

---

[25] Wikipedia Contributors. "Insulin Resistance." *Wikipedia, the Free Encyclopedia.* Wikipedia, the Free Encyclopedia, retrieved January 1, 2018, from https://en.wikipedia.org/wiki/Insulin_resistance.

[26] Mayo Clinic Staff. "Diabetes and Alzheimer's Linked." Mayo Clinic. Retrieved January 2, 2018, from https://www.mayoclinic.org/diseases-conditions/alzheimers-disease/in-depth/diabetes-and-alzheimers/art-20046987.

for Alzheimer's disease, but its mechanism appears to be different from insulin issues.)

The best diets for brain health

There are currently three diets getting attention from neurologists and the Alzheimer's expert community, and all have their supporters. They're really not that much different from each other. They tend to emphasize green leafy vegetables (especially spinach), fish, poultry, tree nuts, olive oil, beans, whole grain bread, and certain berries (notably blueberries and strawberries). They avoid red meat, and some avoid cheese, butter, and stick margarine.

Some Alzheimer's research has focused on the benefit of antioxidants in prevention and care for Alzheimer's, so diets thought to be beneficial to Alzheimer's patients emphasize blueberries, strawberries, tree nuts[27], olive oil, and other nutrients thought to fight oxidation damage in the brain related to Alzheimer's. Do they? My research of the available literature leads me to this conclusion: some. I suspect they might not help with Alzheimer's nearly as much as one would think from the hype because I don't believe the studies supporting their use have adequately controlled for physical exercise. Generally, people who eat well tend to be people who get exercise. On the other hand, people who eat good diets will better control the Alzheimer's disease risk factors of insulin resistance, type 2 diabetes, and obesity.

---

[27] I eat a lot of peanuts. I have read that peanuts are okay to eat, but they neither help nor hurt brain health in the manner of tree nuts.

You can find plenty of resources online to tell you how to implement these diets. The following outlines the diets and says a little about what distinguishes them. I'm listing them here in order of their favorability as evaluated by *U.S. News and World Reports.*[28]

The DASH diet: DASH stands for "Dietary Approaches to Stop Hypertension." It was developed and studied epidemiologically during the 1990s under the sponsorship of the U.S. National Institute of Health, and the work was carried out jointly by several prominent American medical research institutions. Its goal is to reduce blood pressure and so reduce the various cardiovascular diseases. Therefore, one emphasis is on the reduction of salt intake. What's good for the heart is also good for the brain, so the DASH diet comes along as an asset for maintaining brain health.

The DASH diet is rich in fruits, vegetables, whole grains, and low-fat dairy foods. It includes fish, poultry, nuts, and beans, and it is limited in sugar-sweetened foods and beverages, red meat, and added fats.[29]

The Mediterranean Diet: This is the granddaddy of the brain-healthful diets. The other two diets are variations of the Mediterranean diet.

---

[28] U.S. News and World Reports Staff. "Best Diets." January 6, 2016. In *U.S. News & World Report.* Retrieved September 7, 2017, from http://health.usnews.com/best-diet.

[29] Wikipedia Contributors. "DASH Diet." *Wikipedia, the Free Encyclopedia.* Wikipedia, the Free Encyclopedia. Retrieved September 7, 2017, from https://en.wikipedia.org/wiki/DASH_diet.

The Mediterranean diet was developed through the study of eating patterns in different Mediterranean countries in the 1960s. It was first publicized in 1975 by a husband and wife team of American scientists (Ancel and Margaret Keys), but it didn't get traction in American popular culture until the 1990s.

The Mediterranean diet emphasizes olive oil, legumes, unrefined cereals, fruits, and vegetables. It promotes moderate to high consumption of fish, moderate consumption of dairy products (mostly as cheese and yogurt), moderate wine consumption, and low consumption of non-fish meat products.[30]

The MIND diet: In the MIND diet, we have a synthesis of the Mediterranean and DASH diets. MIND is the acronym for "Mediterranean-DASH Intervention for Neurodegenerative Delay." Where the other two diets focused on cardiovascular health, the MIND diet is explicitly for brain health.

The MIND diet was developed by Martha Clare Morris, a nutritional epidemiologist at Rush University Medical Center in Chicago. Morris's research team followed 923 subjects over an average of 4.5 years, evaluating their diets against their cognitive health. They claim that their research controlled for exercise and other external factors, but I read that there is some controversy over how effectively that was done. For example, the researchers said that one can

---

[30] Wikipedia Contributors. "Mediterranean diet." *Wikipedia, the Free Encyclopedia*. Wikipedia, the Free Encyclopedia. Retrieved September 7, 2017, from https://en.wikipedia.org/wiki/Mediterranean_diet.

occasionally deviate from the MIND diet without losing the benefit to the brain, but some believe this suggests that uncontrolled factors other than diet may have been at work in the study population (such as exercise).

The MIND diet emphasizes eating from 10 brain-healthful food groups: green leafy vegetables (in particular), all other vegetables, nuts, berries, beans, whole grains, fish, poultry, olive oil, and wine. It avoids foods from the five unhealthy groups: red meats, butter, stick margarine, cheeses, pastries and sweets, and fried or fast food. Notably, it reduces the recommended consumption of fish to once per week, and it includes additional praise for blueberries.

The MIND diet includes consumption of a glass of wine per day, but I don't drink. I read that the element in wine that aids in brain health is also in blueberries and strawberries, so I count on blueberries in my diet to cover my wine deficit. [31]

The importance of body weight

Obesity is a risk factor for Alzheimer's and a lot of other bad things. (The same goes for smoking.) If you have a weight problem, and you intend to do something about cognitive decline, your first priority is to get your weight down. If you have diabetes, work with your doctor on this because diabetes is also a risk factor for Alzheimer's disease.

---

[31] U.S. News and World Reports Staff. "MIND Diet: What to Know." January 6, 2016. *U.S. News & World Report.* Retrieved September 7, 2017, from http://health.usnews.com/best-diet.

In April 2017, the *Journal of the American Medical Association* published the results of a study that examined the relationship between obesity and the onset of Alzheimer's disease.[32] It focused on people who were obese during mid-life and found that these people had significantly increased deposits of amyloids in their brains.[33] The results of this study were consistent with others that found a correlation between obesity (especially in mid-life) and the onset of Alzheimer's disease.

I read that there are several competing theories regarding how obesity might contribute to the onset of Alzheimer's, and they all point to the complexity of the chemistry of the brain. Nevertheless, it appears that obesity interferes with the utilization of insulin in the brain. Utilization of insulin in the brain appears to play a role in how Alzheimer's unfolds, which is the thought behind the insulin study I have been participating in.

---

[32] "Alzheimer's risk factors study calls out obesity in midlife." April 12, 2017. In *CBS News*, retrieved September 7, 2017, from https://www.cbsnews.com/news/alzheimers-risk-factors-study-obesity-heart-health/

[33] I discuss the role of amyloids in Alzheimer's disease in the appendix.

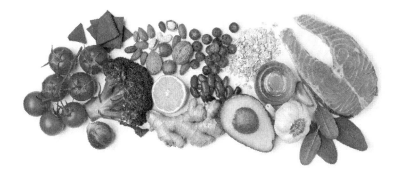

Figure 8-2. Healthful foods help you control you weight and fight cognitive decline. *Photo: dulezidar via iStock Photo*

The importance of good sleep

In July 2017, *Science News* reported on a study at Washington University, St. Louis with several collaborating institutions that found poor sleep correlated with increases in amyloid and tau proteins in the brains of test subjects. The findings were published in the July 10, 2017 edition of the journal *Brain*. The results were consistent with other studies that have found a correlation between poor sleep in people in mid-life with the onset of Alzheimer's disease.

The research consisted of disrupting the sleep of people who normally slept well and did not show signs of MCI. The study found that even one night of disrupted sleep raised the concentration of amyloid in the spinal fluid of test subjects. It also found that there were increased levels of tau protein in the spinal fluid of test subjects who experienced repetitively disrupted sleep. These are indicators of the Alzheimer's disease process.

The study noted that scientists have recognized a correlation between people with sleep apnea and the onset of MCI. (I have been diagnosed with both sleep apnea and MCI, so I use a CPAP machine.) Sleep apnea involves poor quality sleep. Some researchers conclude that poor sleep quality is a risk factor for Alzheimer's disease.[34] My sleep doctor tells me that someone my age should be getting about seven hours of sleep per night, but I have to admit that the older I get, the harder it is to sleep soundly all night.

The bottom line: do what you need to do to sleep well. If you have sleep apnea, use your CPAP machine. If you snore, you likely have sleep apnea. If you think you might have sleep apnea, see your doctor.

The UCLA study

In January 2017, a research coordinator for a drug trial sent me a news release from UCLA regarding a study that claimed to have found the reversal of memory loss in Alzheimer's "for the first time."[35] The research had been conducted by UCLA and the Buck Institute for Research on Aging. The claim was that nine of 10 MCI and Alzheimer's

---

[34] Macedo, A. C., et al. "Is Sleep Disruption a Risk Factor for Alzheimer's Disease?" *Journal of Alzheimer's Disease.* 2017;58(4):993-1002

[35] Wheeler, Mark. "Memory loss associated with Alzheimer's reversed for first time." October 2, 2014. *UCLA Newsroom.* University of California. Retrieved September 8, 2017, from http://newsroom.ucla.edu/releases/memory-loss-associated-with-alzheimers-reversed-for-first-time

patients experienced reversal of Alzheimer's in as little as 2-½ years.

The study was led by Dr. Dale Bredesen who was a visiting professor at UCLA. In December 2016, he gave a talk to the Silicon Valley Health Institute in which he explained the rationale behind the treatment strategy.[36] The talk is available on YouTube. He said that multiple disease mechanisms are at work, and effective treatment must take a "systems approach."

What did the study do? It looks like they did everything even rumored to help with Alzheimer's, including:

- eliminating all simple carbohydrates, gluten, and processed food from the diet, and eating more vegetables, fruits, and non-farmed fish
- meditating twice a day and beginning yoga to reduce stress
- sleeping seven to eight hours per night, up from four to five
- taking the dietary supplements melatonin, methylcobalamin, vitamin D3, fish oil, and coenzyme Q10 each day
- optimizing oral hygiene using an electric flosser and electric toothbrush

---

[36] "Reversing Alzheimer's Disease- Dr. Dale Bredesen, MD." December 13, 2016. In *YouTube*, retrieved October 18, 2017, from https://www.youtube.com/watch?v=6D5aA_-3Ip8&t=3922s.

- for women, reinstating hormone replacement therapy, which had previously been discontinued[37]
- fasting for a minimum of 12 hours between dinner and breakfast, and for a minimum of three hours between dinner and bedtime
- exercising for a minimum of 30 minutes, four to six days per week

Now this apparent success, as documented in the research, is very encouraging. I generally try to do these, except that I don't avoid gluten, and I'm not reinstating hormone replacement therapy. However, there are some problems with the research.

First, there were only 10 subjects. This is not a statistically significant sample. Second, there was no control group. Third, the data was collected anecdotally. The research paper acknowledged these shortcomings and said their research simply pointed to a promising area of further research.

So while nothing on this list will hurt me, I really go to the very last item for an explanation of why this all works: regular exercise. I would bet that a controlled study would find that the secret sauce here is exercise. On the other hand, the hypothesis of the study was that the effectiveness of this set of interventions might be greater than the sum of its parts.

---

[37] I read about one study that found women who continued taking hormone replacement therapy into their mid-80s and 90s may increase their risk of getting Alzheimer's disease. You need competent medical advice on this.

Dr. Bredesen has gone on to do more work, to write more about his protocol, and to offer his protocol publicly. However, some criticize him for moving his protocol into the public arena without the degree of rigorous, peer reviewed, and published scientific research normally required to provide credibility to claims such as he makes.

In his book "The End of Alzheimer's,"[38] Bredesen provides a number of anecdotes about people who more recently followed his protocol and showed reversals of Alzheimer's disease symptoms. Each subject took a tailored array of differing supplements, far more than the five in the UCLA study. But, when Bredesen provided specifics, the subjects' strategies generally shared certain key elements:

- thirty minutes to an hour of aerobic exercise, six days per week
- a generally plant-based diet, often including fish
- a twelve-hour fast between dinner and breakfast
- seven to eight hours of sleep per night
- regular relaxation exercises

Additionally, many reported an effort to remain socially active.

I'm not surprised that these elements, applied together, have produced positive results. However, I would bet that if Bredesen were to throw out everything other than these elements, the results would be equally positive.

---

[38] Bredesen, Dale E. *The End of Alzheimer's.* New York: Bredesen Publishing, LLC., 2017. Print

About fish

Consumption of fish has been encouraged because of the belief that the high levels of omega-3 fatty acids found in fish oil helps with brain health. It is said to reduce damage to the brain due to oxidation. (Tree nuts, such as walnuts, are another source of omega-3 fatty acid, and there are others.) A fair amount of research has been done on this, but the results have been somewhat ambiguous, and the research has not always borne out earlier hopes.

A concern with fish consumption is that the fish may contain higher levels of mercury, and this might more than undo whatever benefit to brain health the omega-3s have brought. However, I've read about research showing that wild salmon caught in Alaska shows very low levels of mercury. Therefore, you will see wild Alaska salmon promoted as a best choice. I stick with wild Alaska salmon.

Regarding fish oil, I've read of some controversy regarding its value. It's often taken as a supplement in the hope of gaining the antioxidant benefit of the omega-3s. However, some studies seriously question whether fish oil supplements do any good. A study published in *Cochrane Database of Systematic Reviews 2016* "found no convincing evidence for the efficacy of omega-3 polyunsaturated fatty acid supplements in the treatment of mild to moderate AD."[39]

---

[39] Burckhardt M, Herke M, Wustmann T, Watzke S, Langer G, Fink A. "Omega-3 fatty acids for the treatment of dementia." *Cochrane Database of Systematic Reviews 2016*, Issue 4. Art. No.: CD009002. DOI: 10.1002/14651858.CD009002.pub3.

Some researchers are concluding that there may be something else about eating fish that's helping, and eating fish is much better than taking fish oil supplements. (I stopped taking fish oil supplements after reading that there is not only a lack of evidence for a beneficial effect but also a correlation between fish oil consumption and an increased incidence of prostate cancer in men.)

Regardless of any questions about the role of fish consumption in brain health, I have focused on wild Alaska salmon (and poultry) for the meat portion of my diet. It took some getting used to because I'm not someone who has always liked fish. However, the potential benefit to me was more than worth the challenge of learning to get along with fish.

Do drugs or supplements work?

There is not yet a drug on the market that has been shown to stop or even slow the progress of Alzheimer's disease. I've been told this repeatedly by neurologists, dementia researchers, and Internet articles. We should all hope this will change soon, but for now, that drug does not exist.

There are, however, drugs that relieve symptoms. For example, I was once prescribed donepezil (sold under the tradename Aricept®) which is supposed to improve cognition. (It mostly just made me very nauseated.) Scientifically, donepezil has been shown to somewhat improve cognition in people with Alzheimer's, but it does not do this by stopping or slowing progress of the disease; it only alleviates the symptoms.

Regarding supplements, this is a touchy area. Many of us with a healthy skepticism about information provided by experts are too willing to form an emotional attachment to less reliable alternative approaches to treatment. The Internet is loaded with the information about "research" that may never have existed and is provided by people who aren't what they say they are. And if we're told that science really hasn't found the answer to what's destroying us, we reach for whatever looks promising.

Do I take any supplements? Yes. Do I think they're helping me? Not really. I reviewed them with my neurologist, and the best she could say was that they aren't hurting me. Some commentators would say that I'm just making expensive pee.

Why do I bother? I was encouraged by the UCLA study that I discussed previously. I don't want to overlook any possibility that something might help.

On the other hand, I believe there is an important problem with supplements. It's easy to take supplements, but it's hard to apply the more important life-style disciplines that have worked so well for me. There are experts who will tell you that supplements help, and there are others who will tell you they are worthless. If they work at all, they are still worthless in the absence of discipline in exercise, diet, sleep, stress reduction, and social activity. I fear that people will rely on the supplements as an excuse for foregoing these necessary disciplines.

Do crossword puzzles and Sudoku help?

Does challenging your cognitive function help strengthen it in the face of cognitive decline? Most of us intuitively think so, and there are companies that sell materials you may use to exercise the cognitive function of your brain. The HABIT study that my wife and I participated in was looking into this, as has other research.

Most of what I've read says that mental exercise does not have a significant effect on cognitive function. You can get better at doing Sudoku and crossword puzzles, but there is a lot of doubt regarding whether the benefits extend beyond simply making you good at these games.

I read an article about what happened when a reporter asked a researcher about how helpful mental exercise was for improving cognition. The researcher said, "People should just put down their crossword puzzles and go to the gym!"

Does learning a foreign language help?

I have often read that learning a foreign language can help stave off cognitive decline. In my experience, however, this is useless.

I began learning Spanish in 2008, and the first symptoms of MCI began to appear a few years later. I continued working on my Spanish all through the period when the decline was asserting itself, even when it prevented me from making headway. My cognitive decline only slowed, stopped, and began to reverse after I began to get physical exercise. In my experiences, at least, learning a foreign

81

language does nothing to help with cognitive decline. (Nevertheless, I have immensely enjoyed learning Spanish.)

One summation

Dr. Frank Longo is professor and chair of the Department of Neurology and Neurological Sciences at Stanford University and is another prominent dementia researcher. In a talk for the Stanford 2015 Community Health Matters Day,[40] Dr. Longo discussed the results of his survey of dementia research literature. The context was preventative interventions for people who had not yet experienced cognitive decline, but the interventions likely carry over to slowing or reversing cognitive decline from disease after it has begun. He summarized his conclusions in terms of the per cent risk reduction. He made the point that, aside from the fact that physical exercise yielded the best outcomes, the quality of the data for exercise is better than for the other interventions. This is because it was easier for researchers to acquire accurate data systematically.

---

[40] "Realistic Strategies for Preventing Dementia; Frank Longo, MD, PhD." June 16, 2015. In *YouTube*, retrieved October 18, 2017, from
https://www.youtube.com/watch?v=SycGjYmZs8M&t=2583s.

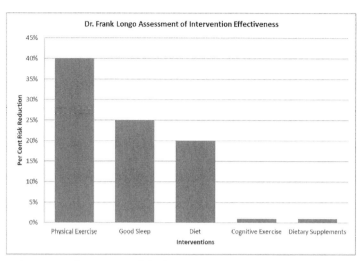

Figure 8-3. From his review of the literature on interventions to prevent the onset of cognitive impairment, Dr. Frank Longo assigned values to the percentage of risk reduction for several of them. While focusing on prevention, these conclusions also likely indicate the effectiveness of the interventions in slowing, stopping, or reversing cognitive impairment after a disease process has begun. The values for cognitive exercise and dietary supplements should be read as "zero."

He also concluded that cognitive exercise (e.g., computer games) and dietary supplements had failed to produce promising results in research. He remarked that his family liked to play computer games, and they liked to go to the health food store and shop for supplements. But no one wanted to go out and walk around the block a few times.

If you can't do the gym

If you're reading this, it's likely that you or someone you love is suffering from cognitive decline. It may be that the things that worked for me will also work for you. I wish you all the best. However, if you aren't well enough to get vigorous aerobic exercise and raise your heart rate for 30 minutes or so each day, you should still do all you are able.

- You should do whatever exercise you are capable of doing. Hopefully, you can walk around the block at least once per day.
- You should remain socially connected with other people, especially people outside of your family.
- You should firmly commit to following a Mediterranean or similar diet and control your weight. It is important to keep your intake of carbohydrates low. Your diet should include fish and some poultry, but it should also eliminate red meat.
- You should do whatever you can to get adequate, regular sleep.
- You should reduce, but not eliminate, sources of stress to the extent you are able. Yoga and other forms of meditation may help you with this.

Of course, you should still watch for a medical breakthrough, and you might consider participating in clinical trials for dementia research. Alzheimer's organization web sites and your neurologist are resources for finding these. (I'm hopeful that the trial I'm participating in will be such a breakthrough.)

Epilogue

T HIS IS WHAT I HAVE LEARNED, and I hope it will benefit you. I wrote this book because I am so delighted with the progress I've made. Beating dementia has been—and will continue to be—a lot of work, but it's really worth it.

What have I learned in my adventure with MCI? I believe that five primary things helped me: exercise, social engagement, stress reduction, good quality sleep, and diet. I learned to eat a Mediterranean diet with fish, and I get to the gym *every day*—no matter what. While I have left the workplace (or so it seems), I continue to do volunteer work side by side with other humans, and I do my best to get a good night's sleep every night. (I do take some supplements, but I doubt their effectiveness.)

People sometimes ask me how I'm able to be so committed to regular exercise and a proper diet. I have not been committed to these things in the past, so I understand the question. I tell them that, for me, this is a matter of life and death. I'm not only fighting for my life, but I'm also fighting for my mind. I'm fighting for who I am. I eat right, and I go to the gym every day, or I will die. When these things were clear, the disciplines were easy.

Please allow me to reinforce what I said before:

- The number one thing that I've done that I believe has helped me is to get regular, vigorous aerobic exercise. I spend 45 minutes on the treadmill every day, no matter what. This generates the BDNF protein that researchers believe repairs the brain.[41]

- I stay socially engaged, even when I, a natural introvert, need to force myself.

- I devote the first hour or so of my day to quiet Bible reading and meditation.

- I do my best to get good-quality sleep every night.

- I have significantly reduced—but not eliminated— stress in my life.

- I eat a Mediterranean diet, and I use diet and exercise to control my weight. I put special emphasis on keeping my intake of net carbohydrates low. In fact, I have come to look on high-carbohydrate foods as poison.

- I fast three hours between dinner and bedtime, and I fast 12 hours between dinner and breakfast.

- I control my balance problems by applying the exercises that my physical therapist taught me. It also helps to close my eyes while I'm on the treadmill. (I do this while hanging on!)

---

[41] As I discussed earlier, some researchers believe this exceeds the point of diminishing returns, but others say I should be doing more. This is what has worked for me.

I am very grateful to the Good Lord that I can drive safely again (although I am cautious and will stop again if it's warranted). I'm also happy to be able to score well on cognitive tests, and I'm glad to be doing better teaching classes. But I think the best thing that has flowed from persistence in fighting this disease is the return of joy to my life. As I could in my 40s and 50s, I can now just stop and think about how well I feel about life. I have many daunting challenges, but my joy has returned. I do not think I feel well because of favorable circumstances; I believe that it is largely physiological. The attack of the disease on my brain robbed me of my joy, but I am fighting successfully to get it back.

Whether someone is facing MCI or they have transitioned into dementia, we all need support. I am so grateful for my loving wife, Amy, who has been standing with me through all of this. I am hopeful that anyone reading this book because they have MCI has a friend or other partner who can provide them with the love and support needed to navigate the challenge of cognitive decline.

This is what has worked for me. You may well benefit from my experience. I certainly hope you will, and I wish you all the best.

Appendix—About the Diseases

IN THE INTRODUCTION, I SAID that I am not a doctor, and I am not a medical researcher. I am just someone who has had experience with cognitive decline, and I want to share my story. I've done some reading on the subject of MCI and dementia, and I've spoken with researchers, psychologists, and neurologists about it. I want to share what I've learned. I encourage you to do your own reading to find out what you need to know for your situation.

What is MCI?

According to its Wikipedia entry, MCI is "a brain function syndrome involving the onset and evolution of cognitive impairments beyond those expected based on the age and education of the individual, but which are not significant enough to interfere with their daily activities."[42] Other definitions consider that atrophy of the brain is occurring at a rate faster than expected from normal aging.

I have a little struggle with the Wikipedia's definition. While I have not experienced debilitating dementia, MCI *has* interfered with my daily activities. If it were not for MCI, I believe I would still be working, even if it was only substitute teaching in the high school.

---

[42] Wikipedia Contributors. "Mild Cognitive Impairment." *Wikipedia, the Free Encyclopedia.* Wikipedia, the Free Encyclopedia. Retrieved September 9, 2017, from https://en.wikipedia.org/wiki/Mild_cognitive_impairment.

I mentioned before that MCI is a condition that can have many causes. I read that more than 30 diseases and disorders can cause MCI. Some of these, such as vitamin deficiencies, can be readily corrected, but most are much harder to deal with. In my case, they said that my MCI was most likely an early stage of Alzheimer's disease (AD) because of my loss of hippocampus volume and growth of the ventricles. It's normal for hippocampus volume to degenerate in aging people, but the process accelerates in AD. The experts are quick to point out that AD is definitively diagnosed during the autopsy, so I'm happy to keep a question mark on this one. (It can also be diagnosed with a brain biopsy, but such a radical invasion of the brain is rarely warranted.)

The Alzheimer's Association tells us that AD is the most common cause of dementia. Depending on the source, we are told that 50% to 70% of cases of dementia are AD. Vascular disease can be another cause, which is called vascular dementia, and there are frontotemporal dementia and dementia with Lewy bodies. I believe that my father had MCI, and it was likely caused by the hydrocephalus that was first identified in his autopsy.

And what is Alzheimer's disease?

If you want a deep understanding of AD or any of the other dementias, their causes, and mechanisms, Google is your friend. I will try to give an overview of my understanding of both the science of AD and how AD works. (I won't try to address the other dementias.)

Again, I'm not an AD researcher, but I did once teach cell biology in high school, so I have a little insight on how the disease might proceed at the cellular level.

AD is normally diagnosed definitively during an autopsy, but there are powerful clues while the patient is still living. Beyond cognitive testing, an MRI will likely find atrophy of the hippocampus and enlargement of the ventricles.

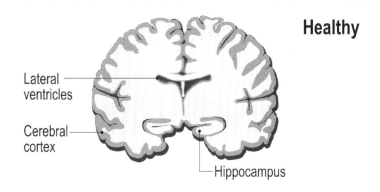

Healthy

Lateral ventricles

Cerebral cortex

Hippocampus

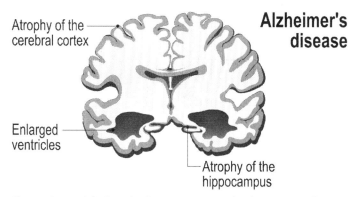

Alzheimer's disease

Atrophy of the cerebral cortex

Enlarged ventricles

Atrophy of the hippocampus

Figure A-1. Alzheimer's disease ravages the brain. My diagnosis was based on MRI scans that showed atrophy of my hippocampus and enlargement of my ventricles.

Also, the disease disrupts the process by which glucose is taken up and used in the brain, so a positron emission tomography (PET) scan can be informative. A PET scan can provide additional confidence in the diagnosis because it maps how the brain is using glucose. (My care team concluded that the MRI was adequate for my diagnosis, so I did not need a PET scan.)

Beta amyloid

In AD, brain cells are dying. Additionally, a protein called beta amyloid is building up on the exterior of brain cells. Some believe that amyloid buildup is a primary disease mechanism—it's killing the cells and/or interfering with the transmission of information between cells. But other researchers I've spoken with believe amyloid is simply a byproduct of the disease process with no real consequence of its own. I have read other authorities propose that amyloid plaques are actually a natural protective feature for the cells intended to defend against microbes and toxins. The idea is that their growth may just get out of hand.

A focus of research has been in removing accumulated amyloid plaques in diseased brains. Will removing amyloid improve brain function by improving the movement of information between cells? Will removing amyloid stop or even reverse the progress of the disease? Science is still trying to find out.

An interesting process has been developed in which monoclonal antibodies can be taken from the blood of elderly people who do not have AD and be given to people who do. This is the basis for the proposed drug Aducanumab, which I discussed earlier. The antibodies destroy the amyloid protein, removing it from nerve cells. However, this very recent success in removing amyloids has not improved brain function—at least, not so far.

One idea about removing amyloid plaques is to start earlier in the AD disease process. As I understand it, trials so far have used people who already displayed symptoms of AD. The thinking is that if the treatment is started earlier, it might be more effective. This is an area of ongoing exploration in AD research. In short, the role of amyloids in AD is unclear, and it needs more study.

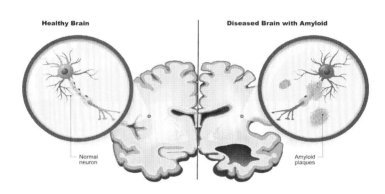

Figure A-2. Amyloid plaques build up on the neurons. In question is whether or not the plaques impede the passage of information from cell to cell. Perhaps they can also participate in killing the cell. So far, removing the plaques has not been shown to improve brain function.

Tau

If amyloid isn't killing the cells outright, then something else is. Therefore, another protein, called tau, is getting attention.

In brain cells (as in most cells), there are tiny, somewhat stiff "microtubules" that, spun throughout the cell, contribute to a sort of skeletal system that gives the cell its structure. Microtubules also help guide the movement of various substances and cell components around within the cell. Normal tau protein exists to help stabilize the microtubules.

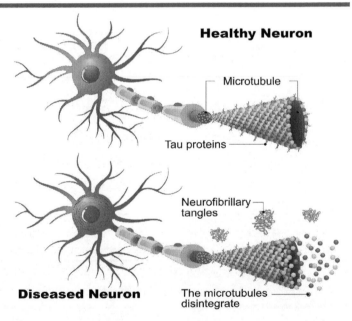

Healthy Neuron

Microtubule

Tau proteins

Neurofibrillary tangles

Diseased Neuron

The microtubules disintegrate

Figure A-3. Microtubules help give structure to the cell, and tau protein supports the microtubules. When the diseased tau protein fails, the microtubules collapse into a tangle, and the cell dies.

But sometimes, something seems to go wrong with the tau. It appears that variation can alter the function of tau and cause it to disassemble the microtubules. The microtubules—and the cell—collapse into a tangle, and the cell dies.

Either? Both? Neither?

So which is causing AD—the amyloid buildup or the dysfunctional tau? Or are these simply events and activities that fit innocuously into a larger and more complex picture? Will stopping one or both of these mechanisms stop or reverse the progress of AD? I'm grateful to be living in a time when these matters can be explored with a reasonable hope of finally understanding the disease process and perhaps finding a cure.

The oxidative damage hypothesis

What starts the disease mechanisms in the first place? Among competing ideas is the oxidative damage hypothesis. High metabolic energy demands, elevated metal content, and limited antioxidant defenses relative to other organs make the brain a prime target for oxidative damage. These are chemical reactions in the cells that occur in the presence of reactive nitrogen and oxygen. Several studies suggest that oxidative damage to cell internals, including nucleic acids, proteins, and lipids, occurs during the progression of AD.[43]

Many believe that oxidative damage can be limited by diets rich in anti-oxidants, such as in blueberries.

The role of inflammation

Inflammation is part of the body's natural response to injury, but it can also cause its own damage. A lot of work has gone into understanding the role of inflammation in both initiating and promoting the advance of AD. Biochemical and neuropathological studies of brains from individuals with AD show an activation of inflammatory processes in the brain. In fact, long-term use of anti-inflammatory drugs has been linked to reduced risk of developing the disease.[44] This is the idea behind diets that avoid foods associated with inflammation.

What are foods that promote inflammation? Here are some:[45]

- refined carbohydrates, such as white bread and pastries

---

[43] Bradley-Whitman, Melissa A. and Lovell, Mark A. "Biomarkers of lipid peroxidation in Alzheimer disease (AD): an update." *Archives of Toxicology.* July 2015, Volume 89, Issue 7, pp 1035–1044

[44] Wyss-Coray, Tony and Rogers, Joseph. "Inflammation in Alzheimer Disease—A Brief Review of the Basic Science and Clinical Literature." *Cold Spring Harbor Perspectives in Medicine.* 2012 Jan; 2(1): a006346

[45] Harvard Women's Health Watch. "Foods that Fight Inflammation." *Harvard Health Publishing.* Harvard Medical School. https://www.health.harvard.edu/staying-healthy/foods-that-fight-inflammation. Retrieved January 2, 2018.

- French fries and other fried foods
- soda and other sugar-sweetened beverages
- red meat (hamburgers, steaks) and processed meat (hot dogs, sausage)
- margarine, shortening, and lard

Is AD genetically determined?

This is a question that occurs to all of us. If one of my parents had AD, does that mean that I'm vulnerable? People ask me this all the time. The short answer is: maybe. Or maybe not.

There is a variety of AD called "younger-onset Alzheimer's."[46] In this variety, the disease begins to manifest itself when the individual is in their 50s, or maybe even in their 40s. It is particularly devastating because it may hit a parent when their children are still young, and it more significantly shortens the patient's life. There are three genes that may occur together and are likely responsible for younger-onset AD.[47] As a result, we see familial trends with occurrence of this variety of the disease.

Fortunately, younger-onset AD is very rare. I read that it accounts for about 5% of AD cases.

---

[46] We used to call this "early-onset Alzheimer's," but this was often confused with reference to the early stage of the disease, not the age of onset.

[47] Graff-Radford, Jonathan. Graff-Radford, Jonathan. "Early-onset Alzheimer's: When symptoms begin before age 65." *Mayoclinic.org.* https://www.mayoclinic.org/diseases-conditions/alzheimers-disease/in-depth/alzheimers/art-20048356. Retrieved January 8, 2017.

In the case of older-onset AD, the genetic picture is murkier. I read that there is a genetic factor, but it likely involves a broader variety of genes. It's likely that there are often other disease mechanisms at work with no genetic root.

There is a specific mutation of a particular gene referred to as the Apolipoprotein E (ApoE) gene. The gene specifies the design of the Apolipoprotein E protein molecule to be constructed within brain cells—a protein that participates in brain function. Changes in the gene lead to a slightly altered version of the protein that appears to participate in the AD process, likely by promoting inflammation. But while having the ApoE variant gene in your genetic makeup is a risk factor for AD, it does not necessarily mean that you will develop AD.

Consumer genetic testing companies test for the ApoE variant associated with AD, so you can know whether or not it is part of your genome—your genetic makeup. The U.S. government shut this service down for a while because it was not clear to consumers what the significance of the gene was. The testing companies must now inform you that, while the presence of the gene variant is a risk factor for AD, it does not accurately predict that someone will develop AD. Consumers with the gene variant are directed to seek counseling from their health care provider. (I had my genetic makeup tested, and I do not carry the ApoE variant in question.)

Can brain injury cause AD?

As I write this, there is a lot of interest in the long-term effects of sports-related brain injuries. This is centered on American football, but it extends to soccer. Some of us remember how the boxer Muhammad Ali suffered from Parkinson's syndrome, which is often correlated with brain injury and shares roots with AD. His brain suffered a lot of injury over many years.

Is it then possible for head injury to set in motion the AD disease process in either the presence or absence of other risk factors? Science is asking that question.

In 2007, the National Institute for Health published an Australian study that reviewed the current literature relating traumatic brain injury to the onset of AD.[48] The study concluded that there is accumulating evidence to implicate traumatic brain injury as a possible predisposing factor in AD development. It noted that there is still plenty of controversy regarding how brain injury could be a triggering factor.

Other research I have read indicates that the later in life when the injury occurs, the greater the probability that AD will develop. While a person's risk for developing AD is increased by a moderate brain injury[49] occurring in their 50s, the same increase can occur to a person who experiences only a mild brain injury[50] in their mid-60s.

---

[48] Ven Den Huevel, Corinna et al. Abstract "Traumatic brain injury and Alzheimer's disease: a review." In *National Institute of Health PubMed* (citing *Progress in Brain Research*, 2007;161:303-16), retrieved September 8, 2017 from https://www.ncbi.nlm.nih.gov/pubmed/17618986.

[49] In moderate brain injury, the person is unconscious for more than 20 minutes but for less than six hours.

[50] Mild brain injury may be referred to as a concussion. The person may not lose consciousness or may be unconscious for less than 20 minutes.

Made in the USA
San Bernardino,
CA